Praise for *Meditation*

"Phakyab Rinpoche's amazing odyssey, beautifully depicted in this extraordinary book, inspires so much spiritual courage, strength, and wisdom. Our deepest aspirations and unimaginable possibilities are illuminated by the radiance of this precious jewel."   — KRISHNA DAS, kirtan wallah and devotee of Neem Karoli Baba

"Phakyab Rinpoche shares with us the compelling narrative of how he healed the injuries he sustained in Chinese-occupied Tibet. Importantly, his story powerfully demonstrates what we now know from science: compassion awakens within us our own power to heal both the mind and the body."
— JAMES R. DOTY, MD, founder and director of the Center for Compassion and Altruism Research and Education at Stanford University and *New York Times*–bestselling author of *Into the Magic Shop: A Neurosurgeon's Quest to Discover the Mysteries of the Brain and the Secrets of the Heart*

"*Meditation Saved My Life* tells us that we can overcome hatred with compassion and let go into healing. Phakyab Rinpoche opens heart and mind with the core spiritual teachings of Tibetan Buddhism in clear, inspiring language. He reminds me that bodhisattvas are here with us and that we can aspire to emulate them to reach our own realization."
— GEORGE PITAGORSKY, author of *The Zen Approach to Project Management*, *Managing Conflict in Projects*, and *Managing Expectations*, teacher at New York Insight Meditation Center, and division CIO at New York City Department of Education

"Phakyab Rinpoche's *Meditation Saved My Life* is a beautifully written, heart-gripping, and inspiring narrative of the courageous struggle of a wise and compassionate Tibetan lama who became a great teacher and healer, risking it all and winning over disfigurement and even death. Read this book and rekindle your faith in the human determination to choose compassion and courage, mind over matter; and ignite your own life."

— ROBERT THURMAN, Jey Tsong Khapa Professor of Indo-Tibetan Buddhist Studies at Columbia University and translator of *The Tibetan Book of the Dead*

"Phakyab Rinpoche is a gem, a spiritual teacher whose infectious, joyful radiance fills every space he enters and whose loving, childlike delight lifts every heart he encounters. His very presence is the essence of healing. This wonderful book is a true spiritual masterpiece, a story of profound healing shared with humility and grace by a master of consciousness."

— RAMANANDA JOHN E. WELSHONS, author of *Awakening from Grief* and *One Soul, One Love, One Heart*

MEDITATION
SAVED MY LIFE

MEDITATION
SAVED MY LIFE

A Tibetan Lama and the
Healing Power of the Mind

PHAKYAB RINPOCHE
Sofia Stril-Rever

*Translated from the French by
Claire Belden Webster*

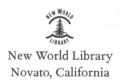

New World Library
Novato, California

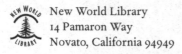

New World Library
14 Pamaron Way
Novato, California 94949

Translation from the French-language edition of LA MÉDITATION M'A SAUVÉ by Phakyab Rinpoché & Sofia Stril-Rever. Copyright © 2014 LE CHERCHE MIDI ÉDITEUR, 23 rue du Cherche-Midi, 75006 Paris.

Text design by Tona Pearce Myers

Library of Congress Cataloging-in-Publication Data
Names: Bstan-'dzin-rgya-mtsho, Dalai Lama XIV, 1935- author.
Title: Meditation saved my life : a Tibetan Lama and the healing power of the mind / Phakyab Rinpoche, Sofia Stril-Rever.
Other titles: Mâeditation m'a sauvâe. English
Description: Novato, CA : New World Library, 2017.
Identifiers: LCCN 2016053842 (print) | LCCN 2017009105 (ebook) | ISBN 9781608684625 (alk. paper) | ISBN 9781608684632 (Ebook)
Subjects: LCSH: Bstan-'dzin-rgya-mtsho, Dalai Lama XIV, 1935- | Meditation—Therapeutic use. | Meditation—Buddhism. | Spiritual healing. | Dalai lamas—Biography.
Classification: LCC BQ7935.B777 A3 2017 (print) | LCC BQ7935.B777 (ebook) DDC 294.3/923092—dc23
LC record available at https://lccn.loc.gov/2016053842.

First English-language printing, April 2017
ISBN 978-1-60868-462-5
Ebook ISBN 978-1-60868-463-2
Printed in Canada on 100% postconsumer-waste recycled paper

New World Library is proud to be a Gold Certified Environmentally Responsible Publisher. Publisher certification awarded by Green Press Initiative. www.greenpressinitiative.org

10   9   8   7   6   5   4   3

CONTENTS

Book Two: May Everyone Hear What They Need to Awaken

BOOK ONE

MY REMARKABLE RECOVERY

The Story of Phakyab Rinpoche
as told to and written by Sofia Stril-Rever

PART ONE

WHEN IRON BIRDS FLY

The natural freedom of samsara and nirvana is like a children's game:
People of Tingri, have a mind without any aims.

— PADAMPA SANGYE

My Fate Is Sealed

NOVEMBER 23, 2003. Since the beginning of the afternoon, flashes of lightning have pierced the sky. It is night in broad daylight in Manhattan. Then, under a lid of clouds, like a fateful sign, the sun breaks through the darkness of my hospital room. Its gaze uncovers my suffering like a wide-open eye within the rough weather storming against the skyscrapers of New York. I struggle to sit up; my trunk is strapped into an arched metal corset. It clasps me in its rigid grip like a turtle's shell — one mutated with aluminum and polypropylene scales and sometimes so tight I am suffocating. Yet this physical torture is necessary to support my vertebrae, which are being eaten away by spinal tuberculosis.

I close my eyes and breathe deeply to try to control the pain. I have shooting pains in my back and, at close intervals, tearing pains in my right foot, which is deformed by an advanced stage of gangrene. The dressing cannot hold the unbearable stench of purulent flesh emanating from my wound — causing nausea.

The peals of thunder become less frequent. The thunderstorm moves away. A new wave of sunlight floods through the drawn curtains of the window. I happily welcome its warmth on my face. Its dazzling rays carry me far away, very far away from Bellevue

Hospital in Lower Manhattan. I am moving around in the supernatural radiance of the heart of Avalokiteshvara, the Buddha of Compassion, who has a thousand hands. In the open palm of each hand is an eye, so that a thousand eyes carefully watch over the ocean of world sufferings, which he endeavors to salve.

For us Tibetans, the Dalai Lama embodies the presence of awakened compassion on Earth. I recall his face, the sharpness of his look. He speaks to me. Within my mind, he utters every word of the message I was delivered this morning. His words reverberate with powerful conviction and finality: "Why do you seek healing outside of yourself? You have within you the wisdom that heals, and once healed, you will teach the world how to heal."

How to heal?

It is a challenge for a man as sick as I. How can I stop the secondary bacterial infection that has been exhausting my body for six months? According to the doctors, there is no way to cure its spread. They are positive. If I do not immediately follow their recommendation to amputate my right leg below the knee, the gangrene will soon become uncontrollable. I will die in agony. Last week, they formally requested that I submit to their medical protocol and get prepared for an operation. Otherwise, they would no longer be able to handle my case as a patient at Bellevue Hospital. I would, however, continue to benefit from treatments by various specialists as part of the Program for Survivors of Torture, which is managed by the U.S. Department of Health and Human Services. Thanks to this service, former political prisoners like myself are granted medical care or even hospitalization free of charge, in order to heal the consequences of abuse and ill treatment inflicted in countries where civil and human rights are not respected.

The necrosis in my right ankle, the result of police brutality, has been described as "destructive." According to the diagnosis,

the process of decay in the cartilage, bones, and tissues is irreversible and too advanced to consider more-conservative surgery. I
have consulted several rheumatologists. They were unanimous. I
could see fear and disbelief in their eyes.

In the condition I am in now, how can I afford to wait, to
doubt, or to postpone? Have I really understood the seriousness
of my condition or how urgent this operation has become? Has the
interpreter, who translates the consultations from English into Tibetan, given me full information? Despite the many alarmist recommendations, an inner voice tells me not to accept amputation.

To clarify my mind, I wrote my question to the Dalai Lama.
The answer I have just received from him reinforces what I instinctively feel. I will no longer wait. As soon as possible, I will
tell the orthopedic surgeon that I have made my decision. I will
then bid farewell to the nursing team that has so benevolently
taken care of me since May 2003.

My fate is sealed.

I Grew Up with Growing Mountains

Flying toward the Unknown

Saturday, April 26, 2003. The Royal Jordanian plane cuts through the veil of heat that shrouds the city of Delhi in the early morning. It gains altitude and, for ten minutes or so, flies along an arch of mountains blocking the distant skyline. Seen from the sky, the rocky barrier seems to recede, but its mountainous landscape stands out against India's open countryside of Haryana. It is as if it has been stretched upward by the power of an extraordinary will. These are the cyclopean boundaries of the Roof of the World — Tibet, my country.

The summits draw a white-inked line, like calligraphy on the ochre soil, slicing through the cloudless sky, forming a stealthy track I can follow through the window. Then I turn my head in vain. The message — if message there was — has vanished behind me, as fast as a flash of lightning. I am unable to decipher it. My heart is heavy with loss. I have thrice risked my life and braved this rocky and icy belt. After much unbelievable difficulty, I have struggled up passes more than sixteen thousand feet high, with no equipment, no shoes, no appropriate clothing. I was compelled to walk by night to escape Chinese patrols so that I might reach the hallowed land of India and receive the transmission of the wisdom that awakens the mind to its true nature. Today, I am flying far away, toward my destiny, toward the unknown.

At the age of thirty-seven, I have spent twenty years studying Buddhist scriptures, along with commentaries by generations of Indian pundits and Tibetan yogis. During lengthy meditations, in the secrecy of solitary caves, I have contemplated the loving and radiant basis of the mind that transmigrates into the cycle of lives. But in geography and biology, I do not even have the elementary knowledge of a middle school pupil. I do not know that the Himalayas are the youngest and highest mountain range on Earth, with some fifty summits exceeding twenty-two thousand feet. Only later will I learn that, in the dawn of time, instead of these mountains, there was an ancient sea that Western geophysicists call the Tethys Ocean, and also that scientists believe, forty million years earlier, continental drift caused a fantastic collision of India against the shield of Central Asia. The junction line between these territories follows the uneven course of the Brahmaputra River, which has its source in Tibet, where it is called the Yarlung Tsangpo River in memory of the kings of our first dynasty.

As if under the action of an awl, the successive pressures of the Indian subcontinent raised the seabed of the Tethys, and from its abysses emerged the Country of Snow. In fact, the series of grandiose Himalayan peaks evokes an ocean of gigantic waves, petrified during the climax of an apocalyptic storm and frozen durably under sheaths of ice. Saltwater lakes were left behind by the receding sea, as well as arborescent corals, pearls, and shells, which were highly valued by nomadic people. A profusion of these can be found on the high plateaus. As children, we delighted in unearthing them for the jewelry and finery my mother used to make.

The upward movement of the Himalayas is ongoing today. Topographical surveys show that this is constant and never ceasing, rising by approximately four inches per year. I have felt this pressure of the earth toward the sky. I felt it in my body as a child. I grew up with growing mountains. The wide-sweeping movements of the tectonic plates can be seen in the landscapes where I used to graze my droves of yaks and my flocks of goats and sheep.

I remember vast, serene expanses stretching out as far as we could see, which suddenly mixed with tangled, rugged mountainous landscapes. I also remember the nearby Nyagchu River racing at the speed of an unbridled horse to meet the Blue River, as it rushed toward the Asian lowlands through jagged-walled abysses. We could cross above these breathtakingly high crevices thanks to bridges whose frail wooden roadways swung over the drops. The deafening racket sounded capable of disintegrating the bodies of anyone foolhardy enough to inadvertently linger over these bottomless abysses. The underground convulsions threatened our lives, since we were vulnerable to landslides and earthquakes, which occurred regularly. To minimize their impacts, our houses were traditionally built around sturdy pillars of whole tree trunks. Nature relentlessly reminded us of the implacable law of impermanence by subjecting us to the fluctuation, and transformation, of the elements.

As I fly away from my native Country of Snow, I recall this teaching of the blessed lord Buddha:

> As a star, a hallucination, the flame of a lamp,
> An illusion, a dewdrop, a bubble of air,
> A dream, a flash of lightning, a cloud,
> Consider the world of phenomena.
> This life is as fleeting as an autumn cloud.
> Observing the birth and the death of beings

Is like watching the movements of a dance.
A life is similar to a flash of lightning in the sky,
It quivers by, and it rushes down,
Like a stream on a steep mountain.

The Mighty Body of the World Coming to Life in My Child's Body

What I remember is that the irresistible rise of the Roof of the World is demanding. It appeals to setting new challenges — in a literal and figurative sense — and to transcendence. It asks us to transform these high plateaus into a mirror of the sky, so that the men living at that altitude can devote themselves, body and soul, to contemplating the divine.

Tibet is a land of myths and legends. I have often noticed how similar popular beliefs are to the invisible reality that today's sophisticated technologies reveal. For example, when I discovered the theory of the primeval sea that once bathed my country in a distant past, it was not really a surprise. My grandmother had told me that the Country of Snow had once been covered by water. Above the water, five pink clouds appeared and hung in the sky before becoming goddesses. They ordered the waves to recede and covered eastern Tibet with thick evergreen forests. To the south, they made abundant harvests ripen, while they draped the north and the west with green pastures. Having accomplished their task, the goddesses returned to the sky to create the celestial Kangchenjunga* mandala. Clouds transformed into goddesses who gave birth to trees, wheat, grass, and finally to sacred mountains. The legend of these origins describes the great cycle of water, which fertilizes Mother Earth in the shape of clouds before

---

* Kangchenjunga is a mountain in the eastern Himalayas, the highest of India, and worshipped by the people of Darjeeling and Sikkim.

rising back to the sky and settling on the mountaintops to become a source of life again.

Without the slightest reference to modern science, the memory of the ages of the world was thus passed down to me. My childish imagination was infused with the greatness of nature. My first gurus were the sky, the rivers, the trees, the animals, the mountains, and the plants. I deciphered the language of the universe long before I learned how to read and write. I only studied the alphabet at the age of thirteen, when I became a monk. By then, without the distorting screen of the mind and its interpretations, I had already been introduced to the secret essence of all things. Besides, is it not in the scriptures? The Sutra of the Essence of the Doctrine teaches the following:

> Even if the Buddha is not present,
> Those whose mind is healthy can hear the sky,
> The mountains, and the trees
> Teaching the Dharma.*
> The pure-spirited truth seekers
> Will see the Dharma arising only through the strength
> Of their prayers of aspiration.

The secret that gives access to the deep understanding of oneself, of others, and of phenomena is very simple. It consists in understanding that everything is linked. Everything is interdependent. Everything is unified. I meet many people whose lives are painful because they have not understood that. They suffer from a sense of separateness — failing to realize that the outer world and their inner world were born together. I have always known that universal life is alive through me. My oldest memories are lit up with joy — the joy of the mighty body of the world coming to life in my child's body.

---

*   The Dharma refers to the teachings of the Buddha.

My Native Province Is an Outpost of Historical Tibet

I was born on the heights that overlook the Roof of the World, in the Sino-Tibetan marches of Kham toward the east. Kham, a fortress of ice rising above the foggy plains of Sichuan, gives Asia its most powerful rivers: the Salween, the Mekong, and the Blue or Yangtze Rivers, along with its tributary river the Nyagchu, whose bold waters rush through the valley where I grew up.* Separated by chains of mountains, their slopes densely covered by forests, their meandering north-south courses recall the curves of giant dragons. They roar ferociously, reverberating the primordial tumult of the spirits of water that cut through the depth of the earth in the hollows of breathtaking abysses.

My native province is an outpost of historical Tibet. I am a descendant of the famous Khampa horsemen, who, at the height of their power, defeated Emperor Munzo of the Tang dynasty, extending their domination in the tenth century all the way to the cradle of Chinese civilization in Xi'an, the former capital of Shaanxi. These fierce warriors, their faces battered by altitude, carried on the custom of bearing a gold-and-silver-butted rifle slung across their shoulder, while keeping a short-bladed and silver-sheathed knife fastened to their belt, both symbols of their legendary bravery. The men in my family traditionally tie in their hair a tassel of red threads trimmed with elephant teeth. They also like to wear fox-skin caps and to throw back the right sleeve of their cloaks, the ends of which hang along their yak-leather boots.

Under Chinese rule, Kham was arbitrarily divided into two administrative divisions on either side of the Blue River, the Yangtze. Today, to the west is the western part of the Tibet

---

* These are the Chinese names. In Tibetan, the Salween River is called the Ngulchu River; the Mekong River is the Dachu River; and the Blue or Yangtze River is the Drichu River. Meanwhile, the Nyagchu River, as it's known in Tibetan, is the Yalong River in Chinese.

Autonomous Region, with Chamdo as the prefecture-level city, while the territories on the eastern bank, where I grew up, were incorporated into the Chinese province of Sichuan.

My family lived in a valley close to the city of Lithang, which saw the birth of two Dalai Lamas: the Seventh "Ocean of Wisdom,"* Kelzang Gyatso, in 1708, and the tenth, Tsultrim Gyatso, in 1816. Lithang was also home to two prestigious lamaseries. One was founded in the twelfth century by the first Karmapa, whose sixteenth successor left his footprint in the rock in the 1940s. The other dates back to the Third Dalai Lama, Sonam Gyatso, in the sixteenth century. It was partly destroyed during the bloody Chinese bombings of 1956, which aimed to wipe out the Khampas' resistance to the advance of the People's Liberation Army. Its ruins, and the Karmapas' monastery, were completely destroyed when the iconoclastic fury of the Red Guards later swept through the area.

My best childhood memories are linked with the life of my family, which has peasant origins on my father's side and nomadic on my mother's side. Historically, in Tibetan society, the peasants, called *rongpa*, settled in the valleys and worked in the fields. Their activities were distinguished from the nomadic shepherds, the *drokpa*, who liked to say with a touch of boastful pride: "We are not herded like pigs under the goad. We fly together like birds."

Recognizable by their heavy sheepskin-lined pelisses, a type of jacket, the nomads migrated during the summer to the high plateaus with their flocks. At more than thirteen thousand feet high, the grass is short and far less lush than in the luxuriant meadows of the green hills of Kham that descend toward Dartsendo, "the gateway to Tibet." This city marks the boundary between

* "Ocean of Wisdom" is the literal English translation of the Mongol words *Dalai Lama*.

uphill, our yak and barley highlands, and downhill, the Chinese buffalo and paddy field plains. Our family would take our herds to graze at high altitudes, where the scarcity of vegetation was compensated for by the effects of the strong solar radiation, which increased the nutritional value of plants by accelerating photosynthesis. Isolated within huge areas, the nomads of my family circle kept alive their thousand-year-old traditions.

Kunchok, my father, belonged to a family of farmers who worked a narrow strip of land at the bottom of our valley. The alluviums left by the Nyagchu River made the land fruitful, while the faces of the mountain kept the warmth of the sunshine, creating a natural greenhouse effect. These favorable conditions, along with hard work, enabled farmers to harvest barley, wheat, and buckwheat, as well as some vegetables, radishes, turnips, cabbages, potatoes, beans, and spinach. Thanks to the strong sunlight — provided hailstorms didn't destroy them — the orchards yielded apples, apricots, peaches, and nuts.

My father traded with the community of shepherds living in the pastures. He exchanged his roasted barley, or *tsampa* — our staple food — for meat, butter, and cheese. While swapping these foodstuffs, he met my mother, Sonam Dolma, the daughter of nomads. Our family assumed a double lifestyle. We farmed our plot of land between October and April, nestled in the hollow of the valley in a gray stone house. It was a squat, three-story, rectangular fortress, its walls capped by a gabled roof covered with shingles that were weighted by flat stones. The large and low front door gave access to a barn and a shed. At the back, a narrow staircase led upstairs to the main room where our family used to gather. Long wooden benches covered with rugs ran along the walls; we used these as seats by day and as beds by night. Rustic wooden tables and shelves were all around the room. They were used to put away the copper or wooden utensils and to keep the dishes that stored flour, rice, water, and other ingredients. Later on, when the Chinese government lifted the ban on owning liturgical objects, my parents set up a family altar on the upper floor. My parents slept in the living room, and my grandmother had a room isolated by a curtain hanging from the beams. I shared a big room on the second floor with my two brothers, and my sisters slept on the third floor.

I liked taking care of the animals. In turn, my brothers, my sisters, and I were in charge of taking them to graze in the valleys neighboring our hamlet. In early May, we would go up to the pastures and camp out until the beginning of fall. During the summer, we would move our camp from valley to valley, so the flocks could find enough fresh grass to feed on.

Traveling on the Flanks of a Yak

At the end of April, we were very busy because we had to gather the animals and pack the trunks with all the clothes, provisions, utensils, and various tools we might need for the four months we were to spend high up. The excitement of departure grew as the date neared. After several days of preparation, once the yaks were at last saddled and loaded, the long-awaited moment would come. My father would grab hold of two deep, woven bamboo baskets, which men used at harvest time to carry ears of barley on their backs. He would fasten them with leather straps to the wooden saddle of a yak on both sides of the animal's flanks. Then he would lift us up — my younger brother and me — and settle each of us in the bottom of a basket. Standing straight on our little legs, we would watch the departure of the caravan setting off at the slow, rhythmic pace of the yaks to a chorus of bells and whistling.

How proud I was when I passed my playmates who were staying in the valley! I never had the slightest consideration for Luda, my best friend. He would sob as he watched me leaving, for it would be long months of waiting before being able to go back to the hut we had built on the edge of the woods, where we liked to go and be alone in the world. Boubou, Nyima, and Lotenpa would walk by my side for a while. I would push them away with a willow branch when they tried to throw brambles or pebbles into my basket. Once, Boubou even came with a frog in each hand to frighten me. I cried out in such a shrill voice that my father interfered and drove him away.

My mother — with my younger sister Tsomo slung across her back — and my paternal grandmother rode ahead on little skittish horses, followed by three yaks transporting our tent, some provisions, and our equipment. At the back, my father, my uncle, and my older brother, Tamdin Gompo, would make sure the drove was moving on. We used to take about fifty animals to the pastures. Not all were ours. Some were white and black sheep, goats, and dzo — hybrids of yaks and cows — that our neighbors entrusted to us. Goaded by the rhythmic whistling and the hoarse calls of my father — or Pala in Tibetan — and of my uncle, and surrounded by four huge hounds, the animals formed a massive bulk making orderly progress.

I remember a nursery rhyme that Sherab Jimpa, my younger brother, and I used to sing at the top of our voices. In the plane above India, I smile as I recall the words:

> He who catches the wild yak by its horns
> Is Magchen Rampa.
> He who seizes the tiger with his hand
> Is Saya Pechö.
> He who harnesses water with a lasso
> Is the Zhongthog yaksha.
> He who builds sand castles
> Is the Kara Kugti bird.
> He who strikes water with a sword,

Inflicting it with wounds,
Is none other than water itself.
He who follows the tracks of
a pheasant running along the rock
Is none other than the grass.
The bird that can give birth
Is the bat.
The predatory animal that can lay eggs
Is the weasel...

Standing face to face in our baskets, traveling on the flanks of a yak, we would sing the words each in turn at the top of our voices, while making faces and upsetting gestures. Sometimes I managed to frighten Sherab Jimpa, who was two years younger than me. He would collapse in tears — but he also liked to pretend to be afraid. In those moments, he would curl up at the bottom of his basket, and I had to pull him out. To do that, I would cling to the saddle of the yak with all my might and haul myself onto its back. I would call Sherab Jimpa, hit his head, or pull his hair. I would sometimes slip and fall into his basket. If I was unfortunate and Pala saw me, he would scold me and make me dismount and walk with the animals. That is, until my grandmother, warned by my cries, came to rescue me. She would put me back into my basket while muttering accusations against my father, calling him a child-batterer who wanted me to die from exhaustion! I preferred attempting this kind of trick when Pala was in the process of bringing wandering animals back, but I remember how the fear of being caught made the scheme all the more exciting.

I will never forget the face of my little brother appearing suddenly in front of me on the other side of the yak. I can still see his thin skin, his chubby cheeks, and his well-defined lips, which looked as if they were drawn by an artist fervently carving the mouth of a Buddha. His features were so delicate, his softness so delightful, that Sherab seemed to have descended from the pure land of the *deva*.*Moved by him, I would melt. By contrast, I felt I had craggy features. I was afraid of hurting him, and I never behaved toward him as I did with my playmates, who were little rascals like me. I didn't hesitate to bully them as we competed with one another in jousts. We fooled around and enjoyed games that left us with bloody noses, covered in bruises and scratches, and with torn clothes. But with Sherab Jimpa, I was instinctively caring. I would have given my life to save him without hesitation.

My Eyes Open Up. My Heart Opens Up. My Mind Opens Up.

We would follow the same itinerary for each seasonal migration. Yet our feelings of discovery remained as strong every year. It was a new experience each time and a source of intense excitement. Our little caravan would make its way straight north following a trail along the Nyagchu River. At the beginning, the trail was lined with a curtain of bamboo trees. Then it meandered in the shadow of twisted willows rooted in overhanging cliffs. The trail continued through a forest of oaks, their trunks shaded with a variety of green mosses, which contrasted with the long strings of pale yellow lichen hanging from the foliage. The fern-covered ground was dotted with juniper and rhododendron bushes, with their gnarled branches strewn with flowers of dazzling brightness. As we approached, big silver pheasants would flee surreptitiously, their feathered tails crushing the tall grasses. Rabbits sat on their hind legs, in their thick curly coats, watching us. And the marmots would whistle as we went by, trying to deter us, with their

---

* The *deva*, or gods, are endowed with great beauty and belong to the highest realm of existence.

forelegs folded on their chests and their little round eyes, alertly protecting the entrance of their burrow.

I would wait with some apprehension for the moment when the trail would open onto the edge of a canyon with almost vertical walls, which were hewn on a slope of several hundred feet. The walls formed the pillars of a gigantic gaping door that opened onto such chaotic scenery that it seemed the entrance to another world. The spurs of ice, like glaciers, of the Poborgang range pushed enormous rocks, tree trunks, and screes of soil into the gorges of the narrowing Nyagchu. The flowing river surged violently, sending eddies like foamy lightning to slash the granite banks. The racket was terrifying. Sherab Jimpa and I would curl up at the bottom of our baskets under the sheepskin blankets my mother gave us to protect us from the rain.

Once we left the Nyagchu River behind, the trail wound steeply upward, starting with a very sharp hairpin curve. The yak we hung from always had remarkably sure footing. It never lost its balance, whatever the angle of the slope. With its cloven hooves, it would cling to the rocky ground, which was more difficult for horses. At first, the yak's continuous grunting was covered by the furious spattering of the river, but this faded as we traveled. The river sounds disappeared as we reached the first slopes with no vegetation. Fields of stones stretched endlessly, scattered with sheets of ice on which wild donkeys galloped — the amber-flanked kiang, whose brown-streaked backs were the same color as their manes. We could see gazelles with lyre-shaped horns and blue-gray-coated mouflons, whose enormous spiral-shaped horns fascinated me. Very fearful, the mouflons would leap from rock to rock when our caravan arrived, until they vanished into this mineral desert. Eagles and vultures sometimes escorted us, hovering above the cliffs carved out by erosion.

We would make our first stop in that area. I can still see myself running about with my brothers and sisters as we picked up twigs with which to light a fire. On this, my mother would set a tea-kettle, then we would go pick strawberries and tangy berries, a real treat for us, mixed with the *tsampa* moistened with nettle gruel. Everyone bustled until evening, for we had to take care of the animals and to find the most appropriate spot to spend the night, sheltered by our bags and the piled up saddles of the yaks.

We took off again the next morning at dawn, and by evening we would reach wide spaces that stretched as far as the eye could see. These landscapes instilled in me an enduring feeling of boundlessness. Thirty years have since gone by, and when I dig into my memories, I relive that experience, that outburst of immensity. My eyes open up. My heart opens up. My mind opens up. Beyond what I see and my state of mind, I experience a heightened awareness of my body and consciousness as I live all over again this sense of merging with the greatness of nature. This feeling is deeply relaxing. It's an imprint within of an undamaged earth and sky, of a new day, along with the incomparable feeling of tasting these for the first time.

Having reached these far away fringes, where the sky seems so close, Sherab and I couldn't wait to climb out of our baskets. We would slip out of them with the same eagerness we had settling into them. The meadow would unfold under our feet — soft, fresh, smooth, like the skin of an ocean of fresh grass, exuding innocence. There was no degradation. The land was free from any attempts to claim and appropriate it, leaving it battered. Instead, it was lavished with treasures: medicinal plants, common flowers, asters, primroses, saxifrages, gentians, poppies, downy lotuses, and many others the names of which I do not know. At sunset, the slopes of the surrounding mountains took on a golden amber and Indian red tinge. Under peaks set ablaze, the mountains were corrugated with valleys draped by shadows, with thousands of blue reflections.

The landscape imparted to us overflowing energy. Late in the night, my brother and I would run aimlessly, until we were breathless and bursting with joy. Clasping each other, we did one roll after another until we were dizzy. Then we would stagger back into the family tent. We would fall asleep, lying side by side, carried away by a freedom as big as the sky. I still cherish the memories of our seasonal migrations. I can still see us bound, like twins on the flanks of a yak, going through landscapes of contemplative beauty that no longer exist.

Life's Generosity

This trip lasted barely a day and a half, but it reoccurred several times during the warm season, so that the animals could enjoy new expanses of fresh grass. Each trip was a similar odyssey toward a new world, yet the distance covered — as the crow flies — never exceeded eighteen miles or so. But every moment was enriched by extraordinary sensations, from being in a clinch or struggle with the mighty mountains to the enduring strength of the yak. From its breath, its warmth, the grumbling of its long rumination, and the controlled movements of its muscles, I experienced the very essence of a creative vitality that was beyond me. I liked watching the yak's arched horns on either side of its enormous head, the bones of which are reputed to be rock solid. They seemed to hold the sky as an offering to the spirits of the mountain. I worshipped this animal with tremendous gratitude.

Without yaks, how could we have survived? Not only did they transport us, and carry loads of several hundred pounds' worth of goods for days on end, but they also gave us their meat to eat, the milk of their females — the *dri* from which we would draw the butter, the cheese, and the yogurts. My mother would weave their wool, and with the hair of their long fleece, she would make fabrics, rugs, and ropes. Out of their leather, my father would cut our boots, our belts, and our straps. Their skin was used to make the tent that accommodated us. The rough leather was cut into long strips and sewn around the guts, which would then be filled with wet sand and blocked on both ends by my mother. After exposure to frost by night and to sun by day, these became as hard as stone. Then we opened the ends and emptied out the sand, turning them into light, sturdy tubes that we used as pegs for the tents. We even gathered the dung, which was an excellent fuel.

These animals taught me self-sacrifice, confidence, dedication, patience, and resistance. We owned few things, and nomadism does not encourage accumulation. Our belongings were supposed to fit into the three trunks that we carried with us from our valley to the high plateaus. But life's benevolence was obvious in everything.

On some winter days, I suffered from hunger and cold. Yet thinking of my childhood conjures no feeling of poverty. On the contrary, when I think today of those living conditions, in their very destitution, I recall a golden age when our emotional bond with Mother Earth was kept alive. Nature, in those early days of my life, generously gave our bodies all the food we needed and imbued our minds with boundless confidence. We were anchored in a spirit of abundance and renewal. Though destitute, we endured neither hardships nor feelings of frustration. Thankful for each passing day, we were filled with the inexhaustible beauty of all beings and of the world.

May All Sentient Beings Enjoy Happiness, and the Causes of Happiness!

Tibetan families who migrated seasonally, like our own, had not yet been forced to settle down. Thirty years later, in the early

2000s, they would be. They were assigned to soulless concrete housing developments as part of the systematic mining of large underground mineral deposits, which abounded in ore and rare soils. Fenced in together with their livestock, Tibetan nomads were subjected to an annual levy of a predetermined number of yaks, which was enforced by decree according to government quotas. In the consumer society that the Chinese introduced to twenty-first-century Tibet, animals as well as the soil were merchandised. They were reduced to their market value in a race for profits, which relies on continually producing and earning more and more. Though we are very knowledgeable nowadays, we still haven't realized that mineral resources contribute to the energy of the soil and nurture vegetation. They are like the tissues and fluids in our body. By overexploiting our mineral resources, we weaken the earth. In areas devastated by mining, the grass grows back sparsely and is inferior in quality. Our elders intuitively knew this.

I am lucky to have grown up in a world where life was celebrated as a gift, with people and nature in communion. Since then, pollution has spread across our nourishing Earth, from the water of rivers and oceans to the air we breathe on all five continents. As a result, there is a feeling of profound insecurity. Losing our instinctual rootedness in the unity of life makes finding one's inner peace very difficult.

I grew up sensing nature's energy both within me and outside me. This energy stretched outward from my mind, reaching toward infinity, and it returned to me in the form of vibrations of universal love. Thinking of it now, I realize that on the Roof of the World of my childhood, there was no notion of limits. I was intensely linked with the cosmos. Physically united with all beings, as in our age-old prayers, we voiced these wishes for the well-being of all living creatures:

May all sentient beings enjoy happiness, and the causes
   of happiness!
May all sentient beings be free from suffering, and the
   causes of suffering!
May all sentient beings never be separated from supreme
   joy beyond sorrow!
May all sentient beings remain in equanimity, free from
   bias, attachment, and hatred!

The Roof of the World Gives Way under My Feet

When I was in jail, almost every day, again and again, I would go
over these memories of the high plateaus. They had the power to
free me from the oppression of confinement. It was as if the immensity I had absorbed as a child flowed through my veins as an
adult. By throwing me into a concrete cell, where I could neither
stand nor stretch out, the Chinese penitentiary administration
arbitrarily imposed a drastic deprivation of my movements. But
nobody could stop my mind from escaping into boundlessness.

In the plane, ever since take off, I view limitless horizons from
the window. Ribbons of clouds in the blue sky give shape to a vast
and moving expanse. But I notice, during my first trip by plane,
that my view is missing an essential dimension. There is no experience of the body. I can see, but only with my eyes. I remain separated from the sky and the clouds, the objects of my vision. As a
child, I embodied the sky. I embodied the clouds. I embodied the
mountains, and I embodied the meadows. My whole body could
see. I physically experienced immersion in the immensity of life.

We have flown past Kashgar, and we are leaving behind the
thousands of snow paths hewn into the granite heights of the
celestial mountains of Pamir. Attached to Tibet by the Kunlun
range, they form the western foothills of the Himalayas, along the
Silk Road that goes through Samarkand, the gateway to Central

Asia. I will only learn the names of these places a few years from now. For the moment, all I know is that it is the end of the Roof of the World. At this stage in the flight, I can see it giving way under my feet. The mountaintops and steep slopes will steadily yield to the uniformity of the plains of Turkey, which is washed by the smooth waters of the Mediterranean. I am flying away from everything I have loved. I am leaving everything I have known. I cannot help wondering when I will see the high peaks and everlasting snows of the Himalayas again. When I do, I know the Tibet I return to will very likely be unrecognizable. I am overcome with a great sadness to be leaving behind a defunct world.

The memory arises of my younger brother, Sherab Jimpa. I loved him so, but I lost him in 1998. The night before his death, I saw him in a dream. As I approached him, all of a sudden a ray of light divided his body vertically into two equal parts. White on the right, black on the left. The two halves suddenly broke away from each other and fell to the ground. I woke up with a start, filled with a dark foreboding.

At the time, I was in Dartsendo, in Ngachu Monastery, where I was guiding a Medicine Buddha ritual. All day, I prayed for my brother. In the evening, I had hardly finished when a monk called me. My father wanted me to call back urgently. I could guess only too well the reason for his call. I was delivered the terrible piece of news. My brother had been run over by a truck on the outskirts of Lithang. My father, to make it easier for me, tried to make me believe he was still alive, but I knew it was not true. Sherab Jimpa had left his body and set off for future lives. He was twenty-seven years old.

This occurred in 1998. In those days, the road from Dartsendo to Lithang was very bad. The trip I took lasted more than ten hours, and I remember that, upon arriving at our family home, I heard a cuckoo. It is said to be a bad omen to hear one singing for the first time in the season at the close of the day. This bird, that I loved so much, tolled the end of many shared joys, of the complicity and tremendous fondness that had always linked me to my younger brother. He too had become a monk, inspired by my example. He was an excellent practicing monk who was able to memorize the very long texts of our daily practices. He also had an intuitive knowledge of medicinal plants, and he used to help pick them with the local *amchi*, traditional Tibetan doctors. He was loved by all for being so helpful to our community. For he could do so many things without ever having learned how to do them! He was called on to tend sick animals, to fix a car, to repair the electricity, or to set up the television. He loved being useful, and he had contributed much to the reconstruction of Lithang Monastery.

When I arrived, a meditative crowd was pressing in front of our family home. His body was lying under a tent that had been pitched in the garden. He was dressed with his monk's vestments and covered by *katha*, white silk scarves of bliss. On the altar near his head, butter lamps and incense sticks were burning. My mother had also laid by him his favorite food and drink. Offerings are renewed every day for forty-nine days following death.

The Clear Light of Death

Five monks had already started reading the *Bardo Thodol: Liberation through Hearing during the Intermediate State*,* which guides the mind of the deceased through the states of consciousness of the afterlife. As I walked in, the monks were chanting the beginning of the text, which describes the moment of demise.

For the person who is dying, this first phase of separation between mind and body is marked by different perceptions. First,

---

* In the West, this book is more commonly known as *The Tibetan Book of the Dead*.

there is a white light resembling daybreak, then twilight glows, and in the end complete darkness. This last state of consciousness is that of physical death, when external breathing ceases. This is immediately followed by the appearance of dazzling brightness. People who are used to meditating, and who are prepared for it, can continue meditating after physical death for several days while contemplating this radiant light. It is the meditation of the clear light of death that ordinary people only catch a glimpse of, for as long as it takes to snap a finger. A person who practices recognizing this fundamental radiance — the essence of awakened wisdom — learns how to sustain its intensity. By fading away into this light during death, the person will be freed from the cycle of rebirths. Others, those who have not already sharpened their inner vision, do not succeed in immersing themselves into this clarity of death. They are thus compelled to wander for forty-nine days in the intermediate state between life and death called the *bardo*.

In order to soothe Sherab Jimpa's mind, and to remind him of how important it is to sustain the vision of the primal clear light, monks were reading him the beginning of the *Bardo Thodol*:

> Have you received the teaching of a wise master,
> Initiated into the mysteries of the Bardo?
> If you have received it, recall it to your memory,
> And don't allow yourself to be distracted by any other
>   thoughts.
> Steadfastly maintain your mental lucidity.
> If you are suffering, do not allow yourself to be absorbed
> By the sensations caused by your suffering.
> If you feel a restful torpor invade your mind,
> If you feel yourself sinking into a calm darkness,
> A pacifying oblivion, don't surrender to it.
> Remain alert!
> The consciousnesses, which have been known

As the being Sherab Jimpa,
Have a tendency to disperse.
Retain them with the strength of the mind.
Your consciousnesses are separating from your body,
And entering the Bardo.
Appeal to your energy to allow you to see them
As you cross the threshold, and retain total consciousness.
The vivid clarity of the Light without color and
     emptiness will appear
And envelop you with a quickness greater than lightning.
Don't allow fear to make you retreat and lose
     consciousness.
Plunge into that light!
Reject all belief in an ego,
And all attachment to your illusionary personality.
Dissolve its Non-being into Being and be free!
There are very few individuals who,
Having lacked the capability to attain liberation during
     their lifetime,
Can do so at this moment that is so fleeting
That it can be said to be without duration.
Others, affected by the fear
That is experienced as a fatal shock,
Lose consciousness.

I was too attached to Sherab Jimpa. As he had just died, his
mind was still close. He still believed he was alive and could continue to perceive his family and his environment, feeling he was
still part of it. My grief might have destabilized him precisely
when he needed to be extremely vigilant to free himself from the
bardo. I left the room and fell to pieces. I have since learned how
to control my mind, but at the time, I plunged into mourning. It

was three days later, having overcome the shock, that I was able to take part in the cremation prayers.

Thereafter, day and night, I made *tsa-tsa* with other monks. We mixed Sherab Jimpa's ashes into these clay votive figurines depicting Buddhas. Making *tsa-tsa* is a source of immeasurable merits, which we dedicated to my brother. We then filled trucks with these miniature statues and took them as offerings to the nearby lake Dzogen Tso, the "lake of the sacred cow," to soothe, protect, and bless the spirits of water.

Message from the Sky

On the plane, as I recall these poignant moments, we enter an area of turbulence. My eyes are drawn to a group of clouds. Strangely enough, one of them is shaped like a horse that the wind is pushing toward a mass of thick clouds, which evoke the twin domes of two mountains. How could I forget, in this moment, the wonderful dream I had upon waking on the forty-ninth day following my brother's death?

I was riding on horseback, up in the sky, a magnificent spotlessly white purebred. My mount was as light as a feather, and I felt very light myself. I climbed up the slope of a mountain in a flash, and once at the top, a second nearby peak appeared in front of me. Standing on this peak, Sherab Jimpa faced me. His face, profiled against the blue sky, was shining like the rising sun. I spurred my horse; it cleaved through the air and drew near the summit where my brother was smiling, happy to see me again. My heart pounding, I held out my hand. As I was about to touch his shoulder, he vanished like a rainbow in the crown of everlasting snow.

My horse collapsed. It became a river of tears, giving vent to long sobs that woke me up.... I found solace in this dream. The celestial horse, the snowy mountains, and my brother's face, lit up with supernatural brilliance — all seemed to indicate that he had regained shape in a higher realm of existence.

Today, as I fly toward America, Sherab Jimpa reappears to me in the way I see the sky. The odd-shaped clouds, appearing spontaneously, are a sign that the link between us endures, beyond space and beyond time, in the immaterial web of links that karmic causality weaves around our lives. To my mind, the dream I had preceding his death can be seen as a sign that he sacrificed his life for me. The dark side of his body neutralized some obstacle that he protected me from. Later, when I was arrested, my incarceration did not last more than three months, and I managed to escape. Without him, I might have languished for years and years in Chinese jails. Or I might have died in a state of utter exhaustion, subjected to the ill treatment and hard labor that shatter body and mind. Sherab Jimpa saved my life. We have been inseparable from the beginning of time.

CHAPTER TWO

Ragged Yak

I Apologize to Pala

In ten hours or so, I will be landing in New York City, and a bout of nostalgia overcomes me. I know this flight marks a rift in my life. The wind of karma is sending my destiny to the West, toward the unknown. As the direction of my life is radically changing, my heart overflows with gratitude for my family and for the spiritual masters who have passed down to me the best of what they had to give. From the imp I used to be, they have turned me into an assiduous follower, someone trained in meditation and experienced in the practice of inner energy and contemplative yoga.

I apologize to Pala. Raising me was not an easy task. I was a cunning boy, a scheming expert. Very early on, I became the lord at home, for I understood how to use my paternal grandmother's overflowing fondness and the dutiful filial respect my father had for her. Momola, which is Tibetan for *grandmother*, had suffered a lot from the Chinese invasion. Her husband — my grandfather — and two of her sons were killed in the bare-fisted battles the Khampas waged against the soldiers of the People's Liberation Army, who were equipped with machine guns. A third son died while being tortured in detention, and two daughters starved to death at the time of the Great Leap Forward, when the Peking bureaucrats forced Tibetan peasants to grow winter wheat instead of barley. The seedlings, though prosperous in the lowlands, were not adapted to altitude. They froze, and the harvest was lost. Whole families were decimated. Later, during the Cultural Revolution, my grandmother was unable to escape reeducation sessions, the appalling *thamzing*. Subjected to public condemnation, artificially stirred up by the local officers of the party, she underwent cruel humiliations with dignity. My father tried, by all possible means, to help her forget her painful past and vowed to her his boundless love.

Life's hardships had forged Momola's cantankerous character. She sometimes spent several days in a row muttering to herself. Amala, which is Tibetan for *mother*, was the target of all of her criticisms and, without ever complaining, put up with horrible reproaches. This deeply grieved me, and I was painfully affected by the unfairness inflicted on my mother. I did everything to try to divert Momola's fury. I sometimes succeeded, and the family evening would be peaceful. Then, having forgotten everything, suddenly, the next morning, I would be awoken by the same curses as the evening before. These fits of rage could last several days, and my brothers and sisters would be subjected to them, too. Not only was I spared, but I also enjoyed special favors. Once, during a time when we were hungry, my grandmother secretly set aside for me little *tsampa* balls. She treated me to candies. Now, as I recall this, I wonder how she managed to get them so often. But above all, Momola kept my father from giving me the thrashings I deserved.

I liked having fun at the expense of others. To do that, I joined forces with four other rascals, and we never knew what pranks we might dream up next. For instance, with Lotenpa — four years older than me — along with Boubou, Nyima, and Luda — who were my age — we would take positions on the steep slopes beside the track at the bottom of the valley. Our game consisted in pushing stones to stop the traffic on this single, busy, major road. There was no lack of stones of all sizes all around, and when we had blocked one access, we would run until we were out of breath to block the other. In this way, passersby could neither move forward nor go backward. Of course, people understood that these stones had not fallen on their own, and despite our ploys, some of them heard us laughing and shouting or saw us running from one hiding place to another. Pala was regularly informed of my mischief by neighbors who recognized me. He was a benevolent and placid man, but in moments like those, he would fly into a terrible rage and give me a beating.

When I sensed the thrashing coming, I tried to fend it off by alerting Momola. I would run toward her, and if my father caught up with me, I would shout myself hoarse, hoping she would quickly hear my howls. Then she would run to my rescue, brandishing the long butter churn shaft. I would see her coming out from behind, which always caught my father off guard, and she would start hitting Pala with all her might. Of course, I would not warn him, and he had to give up for fear of being knocked out. In this way, though I was the culprit, he was the one to get the worst blows and endless rebukes. I would run away without further ado.

If, as luck would have it, my father made a slight, threatening gesture at me — meaning I had it coming to me — he would only succeed in increasing my grandmother's ire. Giving Pala a challenging look, she would drag me into her room. It was always the same, unchanging ritual. Momola would gather two or three summer and winter *chupa*,* a blanket, and some of her personal

---

* A *chupa* is a traditional Tibetan piece of clothing worn over other pieces of clothing by men, women, and children.

belongings. She would wrap it all into a big shawl, and with the bundle on her shoulder, she would take my hand. At the bottom of the staircase, Pala would beg her not to go. My grandmother would claim he was a monster and that she was leaving to protect me. He was not to expect her to come back for a while. My father would try to justify himself and ask her to stay. Their arguments always went on much too long for me, and without feeling sorry for my father, I would pull Momola by the hand to go. She would inevitably say to her son: "See, you treat him so badly that he cannot stand staying in your house anymore. You're not fit to be a father! I won't live in your house any longer, not even a second!"

We would edge toward the door, and exulting, I would be on the threshold just about to step out when Pala would rush to block our way. My grandmother would make him promise that he would never again raise his hand against me. She would assure him that the neighbors who had complained were slanderous, that I was the best of children, and that my father's punishments were cruel. I would exult at hearing that, and when my grandmother calmed down, I would go upstairs into her bedroom where she would dig me out some treat.

The Neighbors Nicknamed Me Yak Sheldruk

Momola's overflowing love conferred near-immunity on me. I took advantage of that. Today, I believe that my father deserves a lot of credit for wanting to instill principles into me. I am grateful to him for the resounding spankings he managed to give me whenever Momola was absent. What would have happened to me if, without his authority, I was not made aware of the limits I shouldn't go beyond and of the consequences of my actions? I could have inadvertently wounded people by rashly throwing blocks of stone onto the road. When I was twelve, Lotenpa convinced me to smoke cigarettes for the first time, which made me sick, and we left the flock unattended. That had serious consequences. Several sheep and goats were killed by a pack of dholes. These wild, tawny-colored dogs, which resemble wolves so much you cannot tell the difference, are very cautious and fearful. Had we been more watchful, we would have driven them away with no difficulty.

On that day, my grandmother was unable to do anything. Our neighbor Aitsela, who had lost two goats because of us, stirred up the villagers' anger against us. They did not believe a single word of our lies, and we were discredited in front of everybody. Pala punished me by making me work in the fields, and he followed me secretly. One day, he caught me rolling tobacco leaves into Chinese newspapers to make cigarettes, which Lotenpa carried in the horn of a yak and fastened to his belt. My father beat me with such fury that for several days I was unable to sit down. No matter how brazenly I swore to Momola that I was only preparing cigarettes for Lotenpa, and that I was innocent, my father did not lift the punishment. I am infinitely grateful to him for that.

I am also deeply grateful to Amala. I saw her wiping her tears over my pranks, which did not fool her. Though lying to my father was not much of a problem for me, I felt compelled to open my heart to her. When my conscience troubled me, I would go to her to confess my mischief, and she would help me repair what could be repaired, without saying anything to Pala. One day, I felt forced to confess that I had glued the eyelids of my younger sister, Tsomo, with pine tree sap while she was sleeping near our flock. I felt panicked. We were at the top of a hilly path, and scared out of her wits by not being able to open her eyes upon waking up, Tsomo had run off, completely disoriented. I barely caught hold of her on the edge of a precipice. My mother bathed her eyelids with warm water and butter, but she ended up losing some eyelashes, and her eyes remained swollen for several days.

The neighbors nicknamed me Yak Sheldruk, or "Ragged Yak." By fighting so often with others, and trekking on rocks all day, my clothes, as soon as they were mended, were torn again. I was as tattered as a yak that has broken away from the shepherd and returned to the wild, whose fleece hangs in uneven bangs along its body. To mend my tattered clothes, my mother had to stay up late at night, stitching my pants and my *chupa* with ingenuity. I can still see the soft features of her face, worn out by toil. Her hair, plaited in long thin braids, fell on her shoulders like a silky net and was tied up by shimmering brooches on the side. Her slanted eyes sparkled in the glow of the flickering butter lamps. She would prick her fingers to the point of bleeding with the big bone needles, which she needed to pierce the rough, thick material. She never complained about the extra work I gave her. She patiently, and lovingly, strove hard to mend my clothes while reciting mantras.

I had unbridled energy. Very early on, I knew I was different from others, though I did not understand why. I intuitively understood, though I was unable to explain this to others, that my future would be different. In my innermost thoughts, I was certain life would someday drive me far away, far from our valley, far from my family. I never imagined that it would be on another continent, thousands of miles away from the Roof of the World. I was very young when an immaterial and invisible dimension was revealed to me, one that my family was not aware of.

Under the Protection of the Hawk

It is spring 1971, and I am four and a half years old. With the rising of the first saps of the year, even before dawn, the valley resounds with life. I can hear the calls of the cuckoo, the cheerful cries of the sparrows, the tits, and the thrushes, the songs of the larks, and the merry twittering of the magpies. Red-fronted serins are nesting in the junipers, perched on the rocky slope overlooking our farm. I am helping my grandmother pick up the kitchen, and their quivering trills suddenly reverberate. *Tiyu, tiyu, tiyu….* Their joyfully vibrant warbling covers all others. Pure joy. I stand still, all ears. My grandmother puts down the enormous copper cauldron she is polishing. She watches me benevolently: "The wonderful bird is calling you, my boy. Follow it!"

I run out, filled with joy at being granted this freedom. As I approach, one of the serins with a short, thick beak and yellow-spotted feathers flies away toward the cedar forest. It goes on warbling, flying ahead, as I climb the steep path, guided by its singing. I cross a cliff, climb a flat rocky surface, and get my breath back. There is a stealthy noise, a flapping of wings. Silence. The serin has stopped singing.

I call out for it, imitating its whistle, and venture forward. There is no answer. All around, night is falling fast. I cannot find my way back. A cliff is blocking my way, and I curl up, frightened. The cold cuts straight through me. That is when, in the twilight glow, I see a hawk outlined on the transparent canopy of the sky. The bird of prey cleaves through the air in my direction. Having reached where I am, it flies in circles over my head and lands on top of the cliff. I press myself against the rock face. My fright has totally disappeared. Sweet warmth and a feeling of inexpressible peace come over me.

However, it is a threatening night. The wind rises. It is not long before the sky is streaked with flashes of lightning, followed at sporadic intervals by much thunder. Above me, the rock is crunching. Clawing the cliff, the hawk is moving closer to the edge. Reaching the end, the bird rustles the air and widely spreads its wings. The thunderstorm breaks. There is torrential rain, but I can feel no drop. The bird is keeping a watchful eye on me. I fall asleep, bathed in its aura.

Rays of sunlight on my face awaken me. I immediately get up. The hawk is no longer there, but I still feel its protection. It is within me, in the sky of my mind. Suddenly, I hear the voice of my uncle, followed by the sound of footsteps: "Yeshi! Yeshi! Yeshi Dorje!" Then I hear my grandmother and my father. I would like to answer them. I straighten up and make an effort. But my voice is missing. Though I open my mouth, I am unable to make a sound. I remain at a standstill, flattened against the cliff, caught in a stranglehold of silence. When my grandmother suddenly appears in front of me, she is at first dumbfounded before shouting out a shrill cry of relief to warn my parents and the neighbors who are searching for me.

The thunderstorm was very violent that night, and they were worried. Meeting face-to-face this morning, their surprise is equal to mine. As for me, I remain shut away in a silence that they attribute to emotion. My father is so happy to have found me safe and sound that he does not scold me. My mother is amazed to find my clothes and my hair perfectly dry, while all around me the earth, the rocks, and the tree branches are soaked. I do not say a word about this supernatural night, under the protection of the hawk — a night when time stopped.

I Am a Sage Who Possesses in Plentitude the Manifold Treasures of Desire

During that night, I reconnected with my former lives. It was only much later that I understood this, when the secret of my present incarnation was revealed to me. But ever since then, I have known how to call for the protection of birds. Sometimes in Tibet, it occasionally occurred that some animals were missing in the evening, when it was time to bring the flock back. In which direction were we to look for them? The landscape was enormous, and I had no clue. In moments like this, I withdrew into myself and "stopped time." For me, this expression meant being in a particular state of mind in which I no longer listened to the signals of the outside world, but I became absorbed in the dimension of my inner being. This contemplative state — which I later learned is called *shamatha*, or "inner peace" — is achieved through meditation.

When, as a child, I succeeded in creating within this energy of primal peace, I could suddenly see a hawk, or another bird of prey, looming on the horizon. I recognized them thanks to their noble wingspan and their perfect mastery of the art of gliding, which conveyed full trust. With no obvious effort, they would fly toward me in a supple and gliding way, their wings lying horizontally flat with their tips slightly drooping. The bird would bear down on me, as if attracted by a magnet. Once above my head, it would circle and take flight in a flurry of feathers in a specific direction. Following it, I would invariably find the lost animal.

Fourteen years later, in 1985, while crossing the Himalayas to get into India, I would be saved by birds, hawks, eagles, kites, and other vultures. I would follow them, even acting against the advice of our guides, Nepalese Sherpas, who sometimes wanted us to go the exact opposite direction. Yet the turn of events would show that the birds had led me to the right path.

Since that day in 1971, I have always listened to the songs of birds, and I have made my decisions according to their messages. To hear them, I first need to create vast silence within me. The kind of silence, paradoxically, that is not merely the absence of sound, since the warbling of the birds does not break it. Even very young, I was able to sense that the silence that fills my mind goes beyond silence. It represents the space of consciousness underlying appearances, which shows the always-changing world of phenomena.

When we go deep down into this level of concentration, inner peace contains the essence of life, in the world and beyond the world, within us and outside of us. Later, the words of my spiritual masters would echo this experience. They would tell me that deities could take the shape of miraculous birds to reveal themselves to yogis. Like in Milarepa's song:

> I am a sage who possesses in plentitude the manifold
>   treasures of desire
> And wherever I dwell, I am happy....
> The plaint of the cuckoo grieves the innermost soul,
> Irresistibly constraining me to shedding of tears.
> The song of the lark enchants the ear,
> Irresistibly constraining me to sweet listening.
> The busy cawing of the raven, the companion of the sage,
> Benefits the intelligence.

CHAPTER THREE

Night of Pain in Tibet

As Long as Space Endures

The plane lands in Amman, Jordan, for a short stopover, and I take off for New York without changing aircrafts. It is dark in the cabin. I wrap myself up in a blanket and lay my head on a pillow against the cold pane of the window. The flight will take thirteen hours to reach New York City. Thirteen more hours of sailing in the sky toward the West. I recall a remarkable sign that occurred during the cremation of my previous incarnation, the seventh Phakyab Rinpoche.

He left his body in 1960, at a time when the iconoclastic fury of the Maoists had already destroyed most of the places of worship in eastern Tibet. Our valley was cut off from the world, but it was not spared those blind acts of vandalism. The Phakyab Rinpoches are traditionally *gondak*, holders of the thrones of the Ashi and Lithang Monasteries. These lamaseries, which used to shelter thousands of monks, were demolished according to the Communist Party's instructions, which were conscientiously carried out by local officials who managed to draw some material benefits from that destruction. They would, for example, convert into cash the age-old beams of the structures, turning them into timber for the barracks or buildings of the Chinese administration. First, however, the statues of deities were taken down. Specialized teams removed the precious stones from inside the statues — which had been ritually filled up by monks — along with relics, mantra rolls with fine calligraphy in gold ink, and incense powder.* After that, the diamonds, turquoise, lapis lazuli, and other various jewels that covered the body were extracted with pliers and tongs. The eyeless face, the desecrated body, and the objects were eventually sorted according to their different metals. The gold, silver, copper, and bronze artifacts were stacked into separate boxes. Then columns of army trucks, filled with the desecrated treasures from the Roof of the World, took them via Dartsendo to the foundries of the Chinese People's Republic.

As this was happening, my predecessor was being hunted down by the Chinese People's Armed Police, and he took shelter in the inaccessible caves of the Gompo Nechen massif. All of his ritual objects, books, and clothes were desecrated and destroyed. He carried on his solitary meditations like Milarepa in his cave, without owning anything other than the treasures of his wisdom and his unconditional love for all beings.

Though she endured dreadful torture, his sister never revealed the place where he was hiding. Suspected of providing him with fresh supplies, she was imprisoned so that he would starve to death. The Chinese Communists considered lamas to be parasites, living at the expense of others. They were seen as disgraceful in modern society, and starving them was a sign of patriotism. That did not take into account the resilience of these great masters, who were well-versed in *chu-len* retreats, their ritual fasting.

Chu-len, in Tibetan, literally means "to extract the essence

---

* Ritual Tibetan statues are stuffed with precious objects, such as sacred scrolls of mantras, precious stones, incense, cedar chips, and precious pills. They are then sealed and consecrated.

of." It is the name given to the pills that help through the first days of food deprivation. They are a mixture of pollen and flower petals, to which are added gold, silver, copper, detoxified mercury, sacred earth, and relics. They are also filled with the energy conveyed by the millions of mantras and prayers that are recited while they are being made. For twenty-one days during a retreat, the meditator first swallows three pills in the morning, at noon, and in the evening, then only one in the following days. That is, until the practice gets deeper and becomes purely contemplative.

The yogi's training allows him to radiate from his heart rainbow-colored rays filled with love and compassion in all directions of the universe. This immaterial light magnetizes the basic vibration of the elements — earth, water, fire, air, and space — while concentrating the perfect energies of awakened beings, planets, and the spirits of nature, as well as the wonderful qualities of sentient beings and the world's intelligence. The practitioner visualizes light flowing through his subtle nervous system, just like a glistening five-colored river. This pure nectar of wisdom has the power to sustain the body, filling the meditator with a sensation of bliss and establishing his spirit in great clarity. At the beginning of the practice, it is necessary to be supported by the energy concentrated in the pills. But trained yogis can thereafter do without them because they directly absorb the energy of the elements through their heart.

At the beginning of the occupation of Tibet, the Chinese authorities greeted favorably the news that lamas survived only thanks to their ritual fasting. This was coherent with their doctrine, since in that way lamas were not taking advantage of the work of others. But the Chinese later forbade that practice, saying it was a "disgrace to the nation." Owning pills for the *chu-len* became "a subtle counter-revolutionary crime." They could not be found anymore, and making them became impossible. Since my lineage goes back to the great saint and yogi Padampa Sangye, to whom the practice of *chu-len* was directly transmitted by the goddess Vajrayogini, the seventh Phakyab Rinpoche was able to survive by fasting and by hiding in mountain caves.

For almost four years, he escaped Chinese police raids, and he once stated that his knowledge of longevity practices would allow him to live for a hundred years. But given the rampant climate of terror at that time in eastern Tibet, he felt he was causing unbearable police harassment and brutality for his family circle. Therefore, he decided to leave his body prematurely, and he urged his family and followers to stop reciting Long Life Prayers for him. A week later, he left for the pure lands. His sister discovered his stiffened body in a meditation posture in his cave. She secretly organized his cremation. The people who attended reported that the wind first blew the smoke away toward the east and then pushed it toward the west. These signs are always methodically recorded, for the spirit of the lama uses them to indicate the direction in which his next reincarnation will be found. That is precisely where I was born, to the east of the cremation spot of my predecessor, and today I am being carried away to the West by karma.

Lamas are traditionally called *Rinpoche. Rinpoche* means "precious"; what makes them precious is the process of their rebirth. They are not born like ordinary people, whose unquenchable thirst to live is spurred by a selfish desire for satisfaction. Genuine lamas have reached a level of consciousness that allows them to settle in the heaven of enlightened beings, where there is no suffering. They voluntarily, and consciously, decide to come back into a body for the good of all sentient beings, in order to transmit the teachings that deliver people from suffering, and the causes of suffering.

This is the meaning of the prayer of the eighth-century Indian saint Shantideva, which the Fourteenth Dalai Lama recited in Oslo

when he received the Nobel Peace Prize in 1989, and then recited
again in Washington, DC, in front of the U.S. Congress in 2014:

> Now as long as space endures,
> As long as there are beings to be found,
> May I continue likewise to remain
> To drive away the sorrows of the world.

This Earth, Anointed with Perfume, Flowers Strewn

The plane enters an area of turbulence. Today, I know that air is a
mixture of transparent, invisible, but dense gas and that physical
laws support a plane's flight through the sky. But in the moment, I
have the disagreeable feeling of floating above the void. I wonder
about this means of transportation, which is so different from the
ones I am familiar with — car and boat — that make their way
on tangible things like earth and water. I cannot answer my own
questions, for I know nothing about the air's ability to lift or about
how it is, in spite of what it seems, a solid element.

The bumps become more violent. Water spurts out of my
cup. Children are crying; there is a palpable tension. I instinctively tell the beads of my *mala*.* I call upon Green Tara,† my
patron. Peace settles in again, little by little, and in the sliver of
night seen through the window, I admire the canopy of heaven illuminated by so many stars. In the decade preceding the invasion
of my country, many wise men of the Roof of the World, who
had reached the fringes of wisdom, had the same vision during
their meditations. They saw the sun darkening while a pitch-black
night, a night of pain, fell onto Tibet like a lead weight. Yet at the

---

* A *mala* is a Buddhist rosary, which has 108 beads.

† Tara is a female Buddha in Vajrayana Buddhism. She is considered a mother of all
Buddhas and takes on twenty-one different shapes. Green Tara represents enlightened activity and protection, and along with White Tara, she is the most worshipped.

same time, a vast number of stars rose on Earth, illuminating the surface of the globe. They concluded that the teachings of the Buddha would be eclipsed in Tibet in the near future, but they would not disappear from the memory of people. When the time came, they would enlighten the whole world.

In 2003, these visions seem prophetic. Religious Tibet has died, but the spirit of Tibet inspires humanity. On March 17, 1959, when the Fourteenth Dalai Lama had to escape from the Country of Snow and journeyed beyond the Himalayan passes, he was unable to take with him any of the riches of his palace, the Potala. But he had within the gem of his compassion and the treasures of the age-old wisdom of the Roof of the World. Mao launched fighter planes to chase after him, intending to shoot him in the Himalayan snowfields — to no avail. And when informed of the arrival of His Holiness in India on March 30, the leader of the Chinese People's Liberation Army flew into a wild rage. Mao declared that the Chinese had won the war but lost Tibet. Tibet had escaped with the Dalai Lama, who from his exile has not ceased to radiate his soul throughout the world.

I fall asleep thinking of all that, and upon awakening, I find daybreak shrouded in clouds. Scattered mist covers the shores of the North American continent. Thus, when my eyes actually behold the West for the first time, it is sunrise, in the brilliance of a new day. These hours of flight, now coming to an end, are a transition toward the unknown. Aware of that, I try to imagine the future. But I cannot project myself into what lies ahead. Only a blank page opens in front of me.

What exactly do I know about America? The way I figure the world is not physical. It is symbolic, expressed in the offering prayer I recite every day:

This Earth, anointed with perfume, flowers strewn,
Mount Meru, four lands, sun and moon,

Imagined as a Buddha land and offered to you.
The objects of attachment, aversion, and ignorance —
Friends, enemies, and strangers, my body, wealth, and
    enjoyments —
I offer these without any sense of loss.
Please accept them with pleasure, and inspire me and
    others,
To be free from the three poisonous attitudes.
I send forth this jeweled mandala to you, precious gurus.
May all beings enjoy this pure land.

The First Time I Met Americans

This idealized vision of the Earth is like a hologram in the sky of
emptiness. In Tibetan, the word *universe* is *jig-ten*, which literally
means "support of the perishable living." The universe is a recep-
tacle supporting beings whose existence is "perishable" because
they are subjected to birth, illness, old age, and death. In this universe, there is neither America, India, China, nor Tibet, for that
matter. There are four continents or lands that emerged from the
churning of the cosmic ocean around Mount Meru, the axis of the
world. Human beings live in the south, on the island continent of
Jambudvipa. Their realm of existence — blessed by awakened beings — is blue, and its symbol is the rose apple tree, a miraculous
tree that makes wishes come true and whose fruits shower down.
The inhabitants of this happy land live for a hundred years. This
vision, elaborated in the *Abhidharma*,* seeks to make the mind of
the practitioner awaken to the energy of wisdom. Its truth lies in
the spiritual dimension of an inner universe, which has nothing to
do with the universe we take pictures of from space. This is not

---

* The *Abhidharma* is a treatise that describes and analyzes the world according to the
teachings of the Buddha.

the knowledge we use to send rockets to the moon, satellites into orbit, and planes around the globe. Doing those things requires the external sciences of the material world, such as physics, astrophysics, and geophysics. As I fly, I am aware of the limitations of my knowledge, a gap I still often feel today.

To help monks adapt to contemporary civilization, the Dalai Lama has set up a curriculum in scientific subjects in the monastic universities of southern India. I have not been able to enjoy that opportunity, so as I am about to land on this day of April 27, 2003, I am incapable of locating America — *Ari* in Tibetan — on a map. In fact, I have never even seen a map of the world. In the sleeve of the seat, a magazine has maps. I take an interest in them for a while, but unable to decipher the Roman letters or to understand anything, I quickly give up.

The first time I met Americans, I was ten years old. Two bearded giants were hiking in our valley with their backpacks. Westerners hardly ever ventured there, for access was difficult; we were far from roads and thus from civilization. I had vociferously called for my friends, Luda, Boubou, and Lotenpa: *"Inji! Inji! Inji!"* Meaning "English" in Tibetan, this was the only word I knew to refer to foreigners. We stopped playing with two barely born baby lambs to stare with curiosity at these two unusual characters. We could not have been more impressed had they come from another realm of existence. The two smiling men explained to us, in broken Tibetan, that they were *Arimi*, Americans. We were dumbfounded, barely able to utter a single word in answer, and we gazed at them until they disappeared in the landscape. Before they left, Lotenpa was bold enough to cry out: *"Tashi delek!"** The tallest one, who was very thin, turned around and handed him a pack of chewing gum with a strong menthol taste.

---

* *Tashi delek* means "good wishes"; it is a welcoming expression similar to "hello."

Luda quickly spit out this strange, unusable piece of candy, which could last until it had no taste left. I kept mine for a long time. I would lend it to Sherab Jimpa and stick it under my bed at night. We had been fascinated by the man's gesture when he had zipped down, then zipped back up, the inner pocket of his jacket to take out the chewing gum. We only wore double-breasted clothes and leather or cloth belts. Later that evening, I told my incredulous mother about this encounter. I claimed to have seen an *Arimi* whose garment was fastened by a quicksilver snake. Such was my first contact with American civilization.

The second occurred a few years later. I was sixteen years old and had become a monk. On a pilgrimage to Lhasa, I met several *Arimi*. Emboldened by their smiles, I wanted to talk with them, but they did not speak Tibetan. In those days, I secretly cherished the dream of going to India to study philosophy and meditation in the prestigious monasteries that had been re-created in the land of exile, in the country of Buddha's birth. I thought, once I became a scholar and a great practitioner, I might be able to teach Buddhism in faraway countries like the United States. But this seemed more like a dream. Even if it were fulfilled, it would not be for some time.

When the Iron Bird Flies

Twenty years later, the day arrives. With some emotion, I think about the Dalai Lama, who encouraged me himself to go teach in American Dharma centers. His private office in Dharamsala paid for my plane ticket, and it was through Khamtrul Rinpoche — one of my Dzogchen masters — that I was invited by his students at the Rime Buddhist Center in Kansas City. I repeat the name Kansas City over again in my mind like a mantra. I have a hard time pronouncing these words. I much prefer saying "Kamsas Siddhi," so that the name of this faraway, unknown place sounds like the familiar one of my birthplace, Kham. I mispronounce *city* as *siddhi*, which refers to the miraculous spiritual power of flying in the air, crossing rocks, and walking on water or fire — all the talents that yogis develop after regular efforts in asceticism. These two words, which I cannot pronounce well, are all I know about my destination, and I am unable to write or decipher them. Indeed, I only know the Tibetan alphabet and some Hindi. I am also incapable of writing my own name in a Western way.

As I think about it, I smile at how confident I am. In my mind, there is no place for doubt. Is it innocence or ingenuousness? Rather, I would say that I have developed an unconditional acceptance of the events of life — or what Buddhists call karma. I thus boarded this plane on April 26, 2003, in Delhi, bound for an unknown destination, and I did not wonder for one second how I would survive without speaking a word of English and without money. My fortune amounts to twelve hundred Indian rupees, the equivalent of some thirty American dollars. I have no suitcase, only a carry-on bag with my monk's clothing, some toiletries, and my prayer books.

I clutch the envelope containing the letter of invitation by the Rime Buddhist Center of Kansas City, the letter of recommendation issued by the Dalai Lama's private office, and the official certificate acknowledging that I am the eighth Phakyab Rinpoche. It is signed by the Dalai Lama and authenticated with the snow lion seal of the exiled Tibetan government. These documents are my "open sesame" to the unknown world that awaits, but I only have the originals. Today, I would photocopy them, but on the plane, I don't give it a thought. The Tibetan papers, and their English translations, are in an acid-free envelope inside a colored, brocade cover slip, along with the passport I was given as a Tibetan refugee in India. Stamped with the Ashoka lions, the bright yellow passport is brand new. I also have written down, on a piece of paper, the phone number of Thinley, who is supposed to welcome me in New York for a few days, before I take another plane to Kansas City.

My flight to North America symbolizes the fate of Tibetan lamas. For almost half a century, ever since our country has been occupied, the greatest masters have fled in the wake of the Dalai Lama. They knew their faith would not survive on the Roof of the World, and they went in exile to India, the country of Buddha's birth. At the time, it was crucial to preserve the lines of great yogis and reincarnated practitioners, the only ones capable of ensuring authentic transmission and uninterrupted teachings. Traditional Tibet once counted more than four thousand reincarnations. But since 1959, no new enthronements have been authorized in the Tibet Autonomous Region.

From the very beginning of his exile in 1960, the Dalai Lama has encouraged the transfer of the Dharma to the West. In Dharamsala, he set up a curriculum for Westerners who were interested in Buddhism, so that they could become the first to translate and convey knowledge that had long been kept inviolable in the secrecy of the monasteries. In 1979, once the Indian government allowed visas to be issued to Tibetans, Kundun* took off for the United States. Like him, like the Karmapa and the hierarchs of the four schools of Tibetan Buddhism, and like many others before me, my turn has come to travel to the Country of the Red Men. Thus is fulfilled the well-known eighth-century prophecy of Padmasambhava:

When the iron bird flies,
And the horses run on wheels,

---

* Kundun is one of the names of the Fourteenth Dalai Lama. In Tibetan, it means "presence."

The Tibetan people will be scattered like ants across the
    world,
And the Dharma will come to the land of the red men.

The Dark Age of Kali Yuga

In Buddhist scriptures, such as in the Sutra of the Descent into
Lanka or in the Clear Mirror of Prophecies, we can read the following words of the Buddha on his pilgrimage to Mount Kailash:
"He who, today, is my follower, the Lotus-Perfume monk, will
be, in the future in Tibet, in the country of red-faced men, the
monk called Lobsang Dragpa."

Historically, before their conversion to Buddhism, Tibetans
were called the "red-faced barbarians." Indeed, the lack of oxygen on the high plateaus makes blood rush to the cheeks, giving
them a vermilion color, which is considered a sign of beauty and
good health. Besides, it is a custom among women of the Roof
of the World to brighten up their complexion by rubbing their
cheeks with goat blood.

Oddly enough, the Buddha's prophecy was fulfilled twice. At
the time of the Buddha, the people designated as "red-faced men"
were Tibetans, and this refers to the migration of the Dharma to
the Country of Snow after the Muslim invasions of India, which
occurred in the eleventh century and destroyed the great monastic universities in the Ganges River valley. Today, the story of the
exile of Tibet's lamas has seen the Dharma established in a different
"country of red-faced men" — North America, whose original inhabitants, Native Americans, were also considered "red." The predictions of Padmasambhava are also confirmed in our time, with its
planes — or "iron birds" — and cars — "horses on wheels."

These premonitions fall within the scope of the general

description of the dark age of Kali Yuga.* In the "dark ages" of
the dregs of times — meaning our contemporary world — spirits
are corrupted by the strength of powerful seasonings, substances
that express the corruption of our spiritual forces. Sex and money
are the great obsessions of our decadent era, which in Tibetan is
called *nyidu*, or "the age of remnants." The debasement of awakened energy in the minds of beings leads them to seek and value
"remnants," in other words all that former generations deemed
unworthy and base. Materialism — which the sages of ancient
times found repulsive — is valued so much that, in our contemporary world, it is regarded as a benchmark and the only truth.
As a result, there is a loss of meaning, which leads to the "five
degeneracies" described in the scriptures: degeneracy of life, becoming shorter; degeneracy of times, marked by the waning of
elements and food, caused by pollution; degeneracy of emotions,
expressed in a way that is more and more violent; and degeneracy
of vision, for philosophy gets lost in mistakes. Finally, we are also
experiencing degeneracy with the outbreak of new and incurable
illnesses.

Padmasambhava had warned us that when the time of this
decadent era came, the Potala would no longer be the abode of
the White Lotus lords, the Dalai Lamas who are the incarnation
of awakened compassion in our human world. A warlord whose
face would be marked by a wart (later identified as Mao Tse-tung)
would wipe out the Country of Snow under his iron rule in a bath
of blood and tears.

However, in Tibet, we believe that, just like the sun cannot
be seen after twilight but reappears in the morning, our night of
pain will come to an end in the Country of Snow. On a joyful new

---

* According to Sanskrit scriptures, Kali Yuga is the last of four stages the world is
supposed to go through. It is associated with the demon Kali, which means "quarrel"
or "strife," and it refers more generally to a degeneracy of our civilization.

day, Kundun will reappear in his native land, and Tibetans will be given back their country. On the rooftops of our houses, there is traditionally a skylight. One only has to be patient, and the sun becomes visible again. We are waiting for the sun to come back into our hearts! For the time being, we are suffering, for the Dalai Lama lives far away, exiled on the other side of the Himalayan barrier. In these dark times of great suffering, the United States has become a land of refuge for millions of Tibetans.

Like so many before me, I am about to land in the Country of Red Men. As we enter New York City's air space, we encounter more turbulence. We cross a zone of slashing winds. The wings of the aircraft pitch by several meters due to the sudden gusts, as Manhattan is outlined on the horizon. It seems like I am dreaming in front of this fragile-looking and unreal cityscape of sky-scrapers. As the wind is blowing in gusts, strips of flat land jut out to form the multiple spikes of a starred lagoon on Jamaica Bay. It is the end of my long-distance trip, which traversed over half the planet. During the twenty-some hours of my flight, I have remained very much within myself, absorbed in my thoughts. I have hardly drunk or eaten anything, and I only got up once on the flight between Amman and New York City. I was mostly overcome by a great sensation of peace during this stretch of time, when I could see the Earth and the sky as never before. One thing is for sure: I am not anticipating the disaster that lies ahead of me.

How could I know that I am suffering from a very severe illness?

That I am on the threshold of death?

PART TWO

SURVIVING

———◆◈◆———

Birth, sickness, ageing and death flow
on a river without ford or bridge;
People of Tingri, have you prepared yourselves a boat?

— PADAMPA SANGYE

CHAPTER FOUR

The Program for Survivors of Torture

Safely Arrived in New York City

Once the Boeing aircraft lands on the runway of John F. Kennedy International Airport, I unfasten my seat belt. At last, the trip has reached its end! I wait for my turn to get up, but at the very moment I try to stand, a searing pain flashes through my right ankle. Setting my foot flat onto the floor is agony. Using signs, I try to convey to the steward that I need help to retrieve my belongings from the luggage compartment. I am not sure what he deciphers, but he kindly pulls out my cloth bag, which is made heavier by my *pecha* — prayer books — with their pages held together by little sculpted wooden boards and covered with brocade. I am the last passenger to leave the aircraft, having slowly, and painfully, made my way through the rows of seats.

Safely arrived in New York City, I only have one leg to carry me. I stagger and force myself to overcome the pain as I make my way through the vast halls, which extend into endless corridors. Is it my unusual monk's dress? Is it my unsteady gait or the pained expression on my face that I cannot control? Travelers in a hurry slow up for a fleeting moment and stare at me insistently. Some of them give me a little smile. I can feel sympathy from some, but I am admittedly too strange and too different. Nobody speaks to me. As for myself, I am too distraught by the cramp that is torturing me, as if my leg were being crushed, and I am too embarrassed about attracting attention. I spot a family of Indians who had been sitting in a nearby aisle on the plane. They are inching forward, holding young children by the hand. I try not to lose sight of them. I follow them until the customs check. In front of the security officer, I try not to show any emotion for fear of being forbidden access to American soil.

Once I reach the terminal hall, I begin to realize my lack of preparation for my trip. This huge airport is a foretaste of the United States, a country on the scale of a continent. I don't have the keys to this space, which is laid out according to a logic that relates to nothing I am familiar with. There is no lack of signs, of pictograms, of arrows, and of color-coded billboards. I understand that they form a means of signaling, the logic of which impresses me. All the facilities display a very powerful organization down to the minutest details. Everything meets the remarkable requirements of functionality. Even if I am unable to decipher its meaning, I can sense the incredible intelligence at work behind this reception scheme. Everything seems to have been anticipated, planned, and standardized — everything except me, the limping Tibetan lama, unable to utter a single word of English and seeking his way. I am a living oddity in this system. I smile inwardly at the strangeness of my presence here, at JFK Airport...to the point where I almost forget my pain.

Before my dumbfounded gaze, a huge crowd flows freely around me. Tens of thousands of people probably go through here every day, self-confidently and swiftly, finding their way with impressive ease. As I now know, this airport accommodates an average of a hundred thousand passengers per day. On April 27, 2003 — my first Sunday in the United States — I stop to gaze at these travelers from another world. They seem to move like characters in a film. I have the strange sensation of being a witness to my own life! I have landed in a reality that is so foreign to me that it seems external, as if projected onto a screen! Offbeat and disoriented as I am, I would lose my grip on reality if pain were not violently bringing me back to it. In these first moments on American soil, I am only aware of my existence because of my right foot, which cannot carry me anymore!

Immersed in a delusion that resembles a waking dream, I suddenly hear people speaking Chinese. The shrill and imperious voice of a woman contrasts sharply with the monotonous announcements unceasingly broadcast by the loudspeakers. She is giving an appointment to her interlocutor in a tone that allows no contradiction. What a providential circumstance! Someone here speaks a language that I am familiar with. I stand before her and call out. She gives me an inquiring look, and all of a sudden she understands who I am: a Tibetan lama seeking asylum in the United States because he has suffered tremendously from the occupation of his country by the Chinese People's Republic. She also assesses the extent of my solitude, of my distress. She agrees to help me. I only have some rupees in my pocket, and I do not know how to call the friend who is supposed to pick me up at JFK. Smiling faintly, she lends me her cell phone and dials the number for me, but not without reminding me to make it brief, since it is expensive.

To my relief, Thinley Lekshe answers. He was expecting my phone call. I explain my situation. As I am incapable of setting a foot on the ground, I need him to come pick me up, along with someone to help me walk, and I tell him where to find me. I thank this unknown Chinese woman, whose benevolence makes up for my improvised arrival in New York City. I still think of her with gratitude, and of my Chinese brothers and sisters who suffer, as much as Tibetans, the violation of their human rights by the regime in Peking. I spot a comfortable seat, where I spend over an hour waiting for Thinley to arrive. Still, time flies without my noticing it, so fascinated am I by the foreign crowd.

It takes us four hours to reach Thinley's home in Brooklyn. We change trains and subways several times, since we do not have the money to pay for a taxi. I lean on Thinley, who has two friends with him, Anjam and Atsok. Thinley is tall and slender, and Anjam is short and stocky. The two of them do their best to support my shoulders, while Atsok carries my bag. The hardest part is going up and down the flights of stairs in the subway. Each step is a victory of willpower. This late April is freezing cold. Snow is falling in thick flakes. I discover with some astonishment that salt has been sprinkled on the sidewalks and on the roads. I shiver under my clothes, which are more suitable for the hundred-degree warm season in India. My ears are buzzing with pain. I need to stop several times, on the verge of fainting.

Thinley lives in a 180-square-foot apartment where he is putting up eleven refugees. His companions in misfortune have recently arrived in New York City. Without his help, they would be homeless. There is no need for me to explain. Upon seeing me, they all understand straightaway the ordeal I am in. They, too, upon arriving in this land of exile, encountered absolute solitude and the shock of a foreign country. Added to that, I have to face a painful and disabling physical weakness. Their solidarity, and their benevolence, silent but sincere, go straight to my heart. I am so happy to be able to speak my language! Being with them, I find a little bit of Tibet again.

Blankets and cushions are piled up against the wall by the front door, and I am settled in a narrow sofa, the only piece of furniture in the apartment. Thinley and Atsok lend me a pillow to prop up my right leg, which has swollen tremendously. We share a simple meal, based on *tsampa*. These men are not very talkative, as if they are storing their energy to face the day's challenges. I have the feeling that my tragic arrival stirs up memories, nostalgia, and the pain of separation from their families, who have been left far behind. Thinley and Lobsang are from Lithang, like me. They ask me a few questions about common acquaintances. Then, after a brief exchange, with measured gestures matching this tiny space, they silently unfold their blankets on the floor. It is 11 PM, and most of them fall asleep very quickly.

Though I collapse from exhaustion, I do not manage to fall asleep. Even lying down, even motionless, my right ankle is in a stranglehold of diffuse pain. Some of the men snore. Near me, a twentyish young man dreams aloud. He gives cries of fright. Apparently, he is a former political prisoner and has experienced Chinese prisons and camps. These nightmares last long after incarceration ends. People often remain haunted by the memory of the atrocities and of the degrading and humiliating treatment. The violation of human dignity is so horrible, so painful, that few words can express it.

A bell wakes me with a start. It is 4:30 AM; Tsultrim and Kalsang get ready in the dark. Depending on their departure time, each person settles as near as possible to the door. The first ones to leave the apartment need three hours to reach the company they work for, cleaning windows of skyscrapers. Over the next two hours, the rest of the men get up one after the other. At 7 AM, the premises are empty. Thinley, who is the last to leave — he is a blue-collar worker at a building site — leaves me some bread, a bowl of *tsampa*, and a thermos of tea. The swelling on my leg has not reduced, and I have violent fits of shooting pain. It is so difficult for me to set my right foot on the floor that I prefer crawling on my knees to get to the sink adjacent to the bathroom, which is only a few feet away.

I want to remain optimistic and believe that this will not last. I have been suffering from chronic pain in my right ankle for three years. This time it's more violent than usual, and unfortunately it occurs when I need all my strength. But why wouldn't it wear off like the times before? It is just a question of time and patience. By the end of the week, everything should be all right. I tell myself that I will consult American doctors as soon as I arrive in Kansas City. They will know how to diagnose what is wrong and help heal me.

In my life, I have already suffered hardships. Poverty, starvation, illness, blows, and mental and physical torture in prison. I have already come close to death many times, in particular while crossing the Himalayas on foot, with no equipment. Each of these traumatic circumstances tested my physical and psychological limits. Thanks to Tibetan culture, and its belief in karmic causality, I have succeeded in bearing the unacceptable, such as the barbarity of my imprisonment and the tortures I suffered. I have never gone astray in the psychological twists and turns of victimization — which shifts responsibility onto others — and so life's hardships have strengthened my resilience. At the age of thirty-seven, I have experienced adversity and developed a non-fearful state of mind. At least, that is my conviction. So, in a spirit of optimism, this is how I spend my first days in New York City.

In Thinley's Apartment in Brooklyn

Why would my situation be different this time?

The pain does not subside. Thinley gives me some anti-inflammatory and analgesic pills, which a dentist has prescribed for a toothache. They provide only momentary relief. The feeling of being torn inside comes back very quickly. One week goes by, then a second. I do not go out. My companions bring back food, and I fix their evening meal. Within the confines of these four walls, I can feel the energy of the surrounding city, which I only caught a glimpse of upon arriving, the rows of breathtaking skyscrapers lined along a grid of straight streets.

Thinley lives on the first floor of an average fifteen-story building on Franklin Avenue in Brooklyn. From the single window, I can see only walls surrounded by other walls. They are interspersed with white-latticed sash windows. Metallic staircases zigzag along the façades, livening the straight angles. A blind wall across the street is covered with layers of ink-black dust. Pollution has created carbon downstrokes and upstrokes, clinging onto the façade like a page of writing. For the inhabitants, who do not see it anymore, this wall is an open book describing the dark era of the early twenty-first century. I gaze at this "dark and peaceful guru," which is a Tibetan phrase for our scriptures, since they are the silent masters who never get angry. What can it teach me?

To glimpse a fragment of sky, I have to stick my head out of the tiny window. My perception of the environment is limited to noises and sounds, and I learn how to decipher the soundscape as if I were blind. At regular intervals, the rumbling of the subway shakes the floors, the windows, and the walls. The shrill sirens of police cars and fire engines tear along, piercing day and night at all times. When sirens ring out, together with the vibration of the planes and helicopters cutting across the New York sky, it reminds me of the fury of extreme winds. I have heard it howling like that high up, charging the Himalayan spurs and causing landslides and icy snowfalls, furiously uprooted from the icy waterfalls of the seracs.

The rhythm of cars and buses driving by hardly slackens between 10 PM and 5 AM. In the building, with the elevators going up and down, there is the continuous noise of a pulley. I can also hear voices speaking an incomprehensible language. They rise up from the street and reverberate in the staircase. This English does not sound like the one I heard in India. Voices do not have the same jolly volubility in New York City as in Delhi. They sound very nasal and are punctuated with loud exclamations whose inflections are strange to my Tibetan ear.

I gaze at the air vents on the ground outside with amazement. They continuously exhale grayish smoke, which comes from the depths of the earth and the endless tunnels dug into it. In Tibet, we are concerned about not disturbing underground spirits. Before a house or a temple is built, rituals are dedicated for several days to the invisible inhabitants of the depths. Here, human will has colonized the ground and the underground and also launched a conquest of space. I come from a civilization that has explored the immaterial territories of inner continents and that communicates with the invisible. In these days of immobilization and pain, shut away in a Brooklyn apartment, I discover the hustle and bustle of a giant metropolis, a sprawling outpost of the North American continent. Like a blind man, I travel up and down the city from the inside, with my enhanced inner senses, fingering it, deciphering it.

Has natural life been driven away from these premises? Not a single bird sings. The only sound that is not artificial is the raindrops. I concentrate on their faint plash, letting it echo with my most cherished memories. My eyes closed, my heart sinking, I go back over the course of my life. I am five, I am six, I am seven. . . . There is a heavy rain shower. Sherab Jimpa and I sink into our baskets, bouncing on the flanks of the yak. In a state of contemplation, I listen to the rain with my head hidden under sheepskin, which I tighten like drum skin to amplify its little music. Am I on a trail in the Himalayas or a tarred road in Brooklyn, New York? Sometimes I do not know anymore. There is such a taste of blessed eternity in these moments, beyond the landmarks of dates and locations that we surround our ordinary perceptions with. It was far away. It was before. But no, it is here. It is now. This kind of confusion is a great comfort. It allows the present to expand. Time and space get mixed up along these lines, which water eternally draws, each time it rains, between sky and earth. I savor these moments hanging in midair.

The subway, the sirens, the planes, the buses, and the passersby invariably bring me back to New York, a city symbolic of the West. I have landed here, blown by the wind of karma, which one cannot resist when it blows. I am surprised at feeling the same sensation as the one that permeated my childhood. Up on top of the Roof of the World, you can feel the Earth's momentum. It rises up toward the sky. I felt it very young, and later on, with an unrivaled strength, I felt it on the paths to exile when I entered the undying clinch or struggle with the Himalayas. That is when I experienced the almost unbearable raw power of the elements, which threatened to break my neck, for human beings are vulnerable to their power at such inhospitable and extreme heights.

In New York City, I can feel another — no less dreadful — form of strength: the power of intelligence striving to conquer matter. Here, will is oversized. It carries the city away into a frantic race. New York City, an ocean of busy humanity, never stops. Its implacable swell becomes a series of huge breaking waves. In the little solitary apartment I am staying in, the soundscape reverberates with a bustling echo that keeps the mind in permanent tension. Thirst for action and irrepressible fulfillment. Heightened dynamism. New Yorkers hurry, but where to? To what exactly?

From morning to evening, the city entices its inhabitants. It requires coming, going, doing, acting, making, producing, accomplishing, performing, undertaking, starting, starting again, daring, leading, running, driving, taking, seizing, grasping, holding, harpooning, pulling, drawing, capturing, owning, uprooting, removing, cornering, conquering, robbing, invading, confiscating, using, taking advantage of…all without respite. All these activities aim to grip the material world, from which we expect to draw riches, satisfaction, and success. I can glimpse the suffering of all those who have been broken by the "made in USA" race to perform. Ruined lives, washed up on a shore where you end up dying, simply because you have not been able to join in the American Dream. In this society, where nothing seems left to chance, this dream certainly has its standards and ready-made norms. I understood that intuitively as soon as I got off of the plane.

I am puzzled. I have never ceased being challenged. During my childhood and my training as a monk, I have felt a continuous inner spur to face what is inside. In that dimension, one has to welcome whatever life has in store, be it happiness or adversity. In my unconventional position, what are my chances of adapting to, or even surviving in, New York City?

It is a double question: first, as far as my physical health is concerned, since my leg is affected by an unknown illness, and then, as far as my identity as a monk is concerned. In New York City, I am far away from the lifestyle I chose for myself as a teenager within a monastery.

The Dream That Changed My Life

It's the summer of 1979. I have just turned thirteen. We have gone up to the pastures. I prefer sleeping outside of the family tent, wrapped up in a yak-wool sleeping bag. At that altitude, the earth touches the sky, and the sky touches the earth. With the dampness of night, each blade of grass is mottled with drops of moon in such a way that the meadow becomes a huge starry field, a fascinating mirror of the canopy of heaven. The vegetable fragrance is entrancing. I fall into sleep, filled with the enchantment of the high plateaus.

My mind moves about on a fresh and buoyant day. On the side of a green mountain, there is the outline of a very tall silhouette.

A being of light walks in a golden halo. He is huge. Puzzled, I try to approach him. But he takes long strides, and I have a hard time following him. All of a sudden, he turns around and looks at me as if he has always known me: "Yeshi Dorje," he utters in a voice as powerful as howling thunder, "I am the Maitreya Buddha. Would you like to come with me to my pure land?"

At the sound of these words, amplified by the echo of the mountains, my hackles rise, and my heart pounds. I nod my head in agreement. Maitreya, the protector, walks in front of me on a steep path. He continues walking at a very fast pace. I feel like a gnat at his side and breathlessly try to follow him. We stop, having reached a meadow with particularly soft grass under our feet. It is covered with flowers with wide-open, gold-bright cups. In front of us, a majestic mountain floats on a sea of clouds. Glistening under the sun, the clean lines of its icy vault cut through the crystal-clear blue sky. It towers over the golden palanquin roofs and the terraces of a huge lamasery. Bright rainbows form a canopy of long, space-filling banners. The sky is transparent, cloudless, with no breath of air. I can hear pieces of heavenly music. My heart is delighted as exquisitely milk-white, perfumed flowers shower down.

The Maitreya Buddha turns to me: "Yeshi Dorje, I live here. Follow me!" We go through the archway, across an inner courtyard, whose walls are lined with frescoes depicting scenes of the Buddha's Awakening. A harmoniously proportioned staircase leads us to the door of the temple. Majestic statues of awakened beings, adorned with jewels, are enthroned there. A monk is busy in front of the altar, arranging crystal bowls for saffron water offerings. I can see him from the back. I have never met him, but I know in my dream that this monk is a great saint and an accomplished yogi. A heavenly voice whispers me his name, Je Tsongkhapa. He turns around and asks me with a smile if I would like to stay here with him. The gentleness of his face makes me faint. Catching my breath, I answer with all my heart, "Yes," and I wake up in a gush of tears. I then vow to give my life as an offering to all beings.

Such will be my fate.

Maitreya and Je Tsongkhapa

Under the cloak of stars at the foot of the Poborgang range, a new life started. I became another. Before my dream, I had never heard the names of either the Maitreya Buddha or Je Tsongkhapa. Obsessed by these visions, I ventured to question my grandmother. She was taken aback. She first wanted to know how I knew those banned names, which nobody in Tibet dared say aloud anymore for fear of retaliation. I had suspected she would ask me that question, and I had prepared a noncommittal answer. Momola did not believe me, but she was moved and cried tears of joy. We were alone, sitting on a flat rock, on a vibrantly sunny afternoon. She whispered her secrets in a hardly audible voice. She spoke for a long time, and in the end she held me tight against her heart. The first teaching I received on the path of Buddha, I got from her. With simple and devout words, she brought immemorial Tibet back to life for me.

Buddhas, as Momola explained to me, appear in different times and in different places in the universe to awaken beings. Thus it is that during the present cosmic eon, one thousand Buddhas will come down from their pure land. The Shakyamuni Buddha is the fourth one. When humans have gone too far from their innate kindness, and when there is no longer anything but barbarity and desolation in this world, a fifth Buddha will appear. His name will be Maitreya, "the Lord of Love," or Jampa Gompo in Tibetan. I drank in my grandmother's words, and I asked her if

Maitreya was very tall. "His head stands higher than the highest peaks of the deodars* of the forest," claimed Momola.

She had fond memories of a pilgrimage she had made as a girl with her mother to Tashilhunpo Monastery, near Shigatse in the south of Tibet. Momola had felt swept away by supernatural bliss upon seeing the statue of Maitreya sitting on a throne. She was still filled with wonder when recollecting his gold leaf–plated face radiating with gentleness and power. In his left hand, he was holding the Wheel of Dharma, which represents the Buddha's teachings, and in his right hand, a big vase of jewels, on top of which was a miraculous plant, symbolizing the purity of our natural world. Momola had devoutly turned around the enormous pedestal of the statue of the Buddha of the Future, brushing the metal with her right hand to receive its blessings. The statue's dimensions were impressive, almost ninety feet high, each finger measuring more than three feet long. A thousand golden Maitreyas were outlined against a crimson background on the outer walls of the temple.

It sounded like a dream, and I could read fervor in my grandmother's eyes. For the first time in almost thirty years, she was freely expressing her devotion, which she had repressed in silent suffering since the invasion of our country. Momola suggested we leave one day, just the two of us, on a pilgrimage to make offerings to the statue of Maitreya. Thus, I would create a karmic connection with him, and when he later appeared on Earth, I would be one of his first followers, giving me a better chance of awakening. Dumbfounded by everything I had just heard, I did not dare tell my grandmother that Maitreya had invited me into his lamasery the previous night....

When I mentioned the name of Je Tsongkhapa, Momola's

---

* A deodar is a species of Himalayan cedar tree.

voice choked with a sob. For her, this great fourteenth-century saint and scholar epitomized religious Tibet before its desecration by the People's Liberation Army. He was the founder of the Dalai Lamas' lineage, and he had instituted the two-week Great Prayer Festival, the Monlam Chenmo, which during Lunar New Year celebrates the victory of Buddha over heretical masters. During the first ceremony that took place in 1409, Je Tsongkhapa presented the Jowo — the most sacred statue of Lhasa — with a pure gold tiara inlaid with jewels. This treasure had spontaneously manifested itself during one of his meditations. He offered so many butter lamps that no stars could be seen in the night. The dumbfounded crowd told the story that, having seen suns by the hundreds flashing out of the sacred city, the stars had been driven wild into the ocean, where they would dive every morning. As for the incense offerings, their curls of smoke wove wreaths high in the blue sky and hung huge banners to the clouds.

Every morning during the Great Prayer Festival, Je Tsongkhapa would ritually dedicate this infinite number of offerings with the greatest loyalty to the sutras and to the tantras. He would bless them, vowing to spread the teachings to deliver beings from suffering. Then, during the period of the Cultural Revolution, the celebrations of Monlam Chenmo became forbidden.

Momola could talk forever. The lead weight of a twenty-year silence had been shattered. I listened to her recall treasures from a world that seemed familiar, though I had never known it. I was fascinated to learn that Je Tsongkhapa had dedicated the biggest monastery in Tibet to the Maitreya Buddha and had called it Ganden, or "Joyful Land," after the name of Maitreya's heaven. Had I visited this Joyful Land in my dream? I couldn't believe my ears!

Without catching all of the dream's meaning, I understood that I had been transmitted the precious teachings of Buddha in Tibet by the awakened beings who had appeared to me. When my

grandmother told me about the childhood of Je Tsongkhapa —
who had been ordained a monk very young, and who had been
entirely devoted to his studies — I was eager to follow his example. I was ashamed of being so unruly and of thinking only
of having fun and unscrupulously deceiving others, while he had
been sound and studious since his early childhood!

During the first days of my American exile, I still didn't have
the keys to interpret my dream. Today, I believe that I had to experience terrible pain in order to understand it fully. I first had to
pull myself away from my physical anchors in Tibet and from my
monastery. Then I had to face the reality of serious illness. I had
to dive into the ocean of physical and moral pain with the risk of
sinking.

As a matter of fact, I have never really gotten over the dream
I had at the age of thirteen up on the high plateaus. If one day I
can totally fulfill my vow to serve all beings, body and soul, it will
be because I have remained, on a subtle level of reality, with the
Maitreya Buddha and Je Tsongkhapa. In my dream, the steep path
I climbed — not without difficulty — is a good omen that I will
succeed in rising out of the abyss of samsara.* The very smooth
soil under the grasslands stands for the gentleness of our stream
of consciousness when thoughts exclusively geared toward the
satisfaction of personal wishes cease to trouble it. It shows that
I will manage to free myself from the rough patches of negative
emotions. The flowers, with their wide-open petals, are signs that
compassionate wisdom will blossom in my mind, free from extremes, realizing the lifestyle of people and phenomena, on an ultimate level, in emptiness. And their golden brilliance shows that
I will transmit the essence of the pure golden Dharma. The huge

---

* Samsara refers to the cycle of conditioned lives, which is stamped with the seal of
suffering.

lamasery is a sign that I will work for the transmission of instructions that free beings from suffering, and the causes of suffering. Finally, the music and the heavenly flowers embody the blessings of the dakinis* who have thus taken me under their wings.

I was truly ordained for the first time by Maitreya that night when I followed in his footsteps. Then it was Je Tsongkhapa's turn to do the same, when I answered him yes. The actual ordination I was given later only confirmed this double consecration.

My Decision to Become a Monk

After meeting Maitreya and Je Tsongkhapa in my dream, I became obsessed with the idea of becoming a monk. Finally, not able to wait any longer, I went to see a friend of my father's who was a tailor. He had big scissors, and when I arrived at his place, I grabbed them. I asked him to cut my shoulder-length hair very short and shave my skull. He looked at me, staggered. At first, I didn't feel like explaining, but he insisted, and I admitted I had decided to become a monk. For a few moments, he thought it might be one of my jokes. But he had to face the fact that I was serious and determined. However, he refused to comply with my wish for fear of irritating my father. Faced with his refusal, I started cutting several locks of hair myself, until he agreed to cut my hair and shave my skull, but not before making me swear to tell my father I had done it myself.

Back home, out of my parents' trunk, I pulled a brown pair of pants and a new light beige *chupa*, which belonged to my father but he had never worn it. I put them on, along with a new, white, and well-dressed shirt that my mother had prepared for me for Losar, the Tibetan Lunar New Year. I fitted my clothes tightly onto my hips with a long brown scarf and slipped on my

---

* Dakinis are protective female figures that embody awakened feminine energy.

leather boots. In this outfit, I waited for my parents to come back. Pala was the first to arrive. Once he overcame his shock at my announcement, he strongly advised against becoming a monk. Chinese policies had changed in recent years, but it was still risky. Above all, there were neither monks nor monasteries left. As a child, my father had witnessed the bombing of Lithang Monastery. He had seen how the People's Liberation Army — who had claimed they were bringing happiness to Tibetans — had massacred, while they lay on the ground, all the remaining monks, as well as the laymen trying to save them. Experience had taught him caution, and he was surprised at my decision. Why hadn't I mentioned this earlier? He was all the more annoyed because he had already accepted an offer to adopt me, which was made by a couple of childless cousins who liked me very much. My plans would thwart the promise he had made to them.

Amala acknowledged my father's arguments, but I sensed that my calling made her rather proud and happy. I was the most boisterous of their children; however, my parents respected my decision. I am infinitely grateful to them for that. However, they suggested I seek advice from an uncle, Thubten Tashi, who had been a monk before 1959 and who had afterward been forced by the Chinese to renounce his vows.

Then in his fifties, Thubten Tashi told me that, first and foremost, a monk-to-be had to be able to read and write. He offered to let me live in his home and to teach me some basics of the alphabet. It was 1979, and I was thirteen. A certain political liberalization was occurring following the death of Mao Tse-tung in 1976, and faith and popular devotion were being expressed more intensely than ever. Behind the bamboo curtain that the Chinese had erected, our invaders had attempted to break our hearts by desecrating our beliefs and the spiritual legacy of our ancestors. In the name of an ideal centered on material prosperity, and of modernization aimed at satisfying fleeting desires, they had endeavored to uproot us from our inner continent in order to manipulate us more easily. But the most cruel persecutions were not enough to eradicate the fervor of my generation, which had been raised among the ruins of slandered monasteries and without seeing any monk wearing religious clothes or taking part in any religious celebration. Some very young boys, who like me were barely teenagers, felt the call for the sacred in the early 1980s. Once China's ideological yoke was released, elder Tibetans, those who had secretly remained monks, reappeared to teach the novices. With tremendous enthusiasm, the population of Lithang undertook the rebuilding of monasteries and places of worship. We had no other grant than our fervent faith; no other tools than our hands and arms. We were driven by the ardor of renewal.

The Spirit of Tibet Rises from Its Ashes

Twenty-five of us received ordination on July 6, 1980, on the day Kundun celebrated the twenty-first anniversary of his exile on the other side of the Himalayas. Our temple was a natural and imposing amphitheater, part of the naturally occurring cave network within the white sandstone cliffs of the Gompo Nechen — the "Guardian of the Great Secret" — a dominant mountain close to Lithang. An aura of mystical power permeates this sacred place, and generations of yogis and yoginis have meditated there. A maze of meandering galleries goes far into the mountain and forms a tangle of secret sanctuaries. Nature has thus excavated a raw religious monument full of unlikely archways and forests of pillars that defy the imagination. In the unexpected shapes of cracks, curves, and porches, our lamas have deciphered the most esoteric tantric symbols, thus giving this natural labyrinth a supernatural aura.

We had set up an open-air altar for the offerings of incense that were dedicated to the spirit of the mountain. From an external point of view, according to the logic of ordinary perception, the Gompo Nechen appears as landscape, whose majestic proportions are covered in a mantle of everlasting snow. From an internal point of view, it is the abode of the worldly guardians and of the spirits of the place. From a secret point of view, it is the palace of the united tantric deities Chakrasamvara and Vajrayogini. The grassland spreading at the bottom of Gompo Nechen is so wide that a galloping horse cannot cross it in a single day. It forms a mandala of medicinal herbs bearing the colors of the elements, revealed according to the infallible law of interdependence.

I took my vows in a huge cave. At the entrance, the bedrock is stamped with the footprints of the thirty Pawo — the "heroes" of the "Epic of King Gesar of Ling" — along with the hoofprints of their horses. I was given the monk name Lobsang Dhondup. Lobsang — which means "compassionate heart" — links me to Je Tsongkhapa's lineage, and Dhondup means "he who carries out his wishes." The ceremonies lasted a week. Lamas from afar arrived on the day of the full moon, and we made so many incense offerings that a fragrant cloud lingered for a long time in front of the cave. Floods of blessings appeared in the shape of miraculous signs, which nature gave unsparingly in that blessed time when Tibet was rising from its ashes.

At the Emergency Ward of Bellevue Hospital

After ten days of endless pain in my right ankle, I enjoy some remission. I believe I will very quickly be able to walk normally again. Cohabitation in the restricted space of the flat is made complicated by my disability. We are squeezed in so much that I cannot go to the toilet at night without waking several people. On Thursday, May 8, as soon as I start showing signs of improvement, I call the Rime Buddhist Center in Kansas City. The person who answers speaks Tibetan, and we agree that I will take a plane on Sunday, May 11, so that Thinley can go to the airport with me. I look forward to leaving New York City in two days, and I am relieved at being at last free from this torture.

Alas, on Saturday night, I am struck by such searing pain that I start trembling. It is impossible for me to get up; I am sweating and panting. I spend four days in this situation, with hardly a moment's respite. My leg swells so much that I cannot wear a shoe or a sock, and it turns purple, which worries Thinley. He talks about it with Jigme Lhundup.

This young, thirty-two-year-old Tibetan, arbitrarily imprisoned in Lhasa in March 2001, is the son and grandson of *thangka**
painters. From a very young age, Jigme devoted his life to sacred art, depicting Buddhas of Light in their celestial palaces. In Tibet, thanks to his talent, he was an acknowledged master of *thangka* and commissioned by the big monasteries of the Lhasa valley. That is, until the day the Chinese People's Armed Police decided his art was "counter-revolutionary." Officers seized from his workshop a finely gilded *thangka* depicting the Land of Joy, which he had fervently made for Sera Monastery, and forced him to desecrate it with excrement and wear it around his neck. Then, for three weeks, the officers methodically tortured him. They tried to break his hands in order to crush his soul. For through his hands, his soul lavished on the paintings the blessings of the awakened beings imprinted on the naturally pigmented canvases, which were sewn into brocade frames.

Day after day, Jigme saw his hands dying. Their flesh was decaying, stripping his fingers to the bone. As a matter of fact, two years later, his fingers are still lacerated with purple scars. He tells me about his ordeal with a sense of propriety, to encourage me to

---

* *Thangka* is a traditional Tibetan Buddhist painting made on silk.

seek treatment. He is himself overflowing with gratitude toward the doctors of the Program for Survivors of Torture at Bellevue Hospital in Manhattan. They have given his hands a new lease on life. When he left the prison, he thought he would be paralyzed forever: "I was like a tree in winter. My hands were hanging just like dead branches. Today, it's the beginning of spring. I can feel the sap flowing back."

Jigme shows me, his eyes filled with tears, a little *thangka* he has finished painting, the first in three years. Filled with emotion, I gaze at this picture of Green Tara, the Divine Mother. In the mercy of a powerful vibration of love, I imagine the pains and sufferings of the artist. Throughout his detention, Jigme never ceased calling upon Tara:

> Om, homage to the Venerable Tara!
> Homage to Tara, the Swift and Dauntless Liberator,
> Whose eyes sparkle like flashes of lightning,
> And who was born in the heart of a lotus flower floating
>   on the ocean of tears
> Shed by Avalokiteshvara, the compassionate Lord of the
>   three worlds!
> Homage to She whose face shines like
> One hundred full moons in an autumn sky,
> Radiating the dazzling light of a thousand stars!
> Homage to She who shines with golden-green reflections
> And whose hands are adorned with lotus flowers!

Jigme asks me to bless his *thangka* and urges me to go to Belle-vue Hospital. There, I will enjoy the competence of the care team, free of charge. He offers to go with me.

By Thursday, May 15, the intensity of my pain has not abated, and I cannot stand it anymore. With Jigme, I go to the emergency ward of Bellevue Hospital. Another Tibetan refugee provides me with a pair of crutches, but the trip is a terrible two-hour ordeal.

We have to cross Brooklyn by subway, and we have no less than two changes to get to Manhattan. Then, we have to walk some five hundred yards on 1st Avenue to 26th Street to reach the hospital. I want to put up a good show, so I rest for a quarter of an hour before limping into the emergency ward.

Jigme hopes Rigzin Dolma will be there. She is a Tibetan nurse who advises refugees and helps them fill in the paperwork to be admitted in the Program for Survivors of Torture. If necessary, she also serves as an interpreter. But this morning, Dolma is not around. After we see a doctor, the only thing Jigme understands from the consultation is the prescription. I have to take three different pills three times a day. If there is no improvement within two weeks, the doctors advise me to come back.

I feel the empathy of the nursing staff. Jigme manages to make them understand that I am suffering dreadfully. Unfortunately, I am unable to answer their questions. I can't explain what I feel, how this problem occurred, or when. Upon leaving, I say my first words of English, shyly repeating "Thank you," which amuses the nursing team. I am deeply touched and grateful for all the respect and consideration these strangers have for me. One after another, they have been at my bedside and spent a long time trying to understand my case. On several occasions, they question Jigme, who tries his best to answer with gestures and signs.

I notice in Bellevue, even more than at JFK Airport, the remarkable facilities and the efficient organization. Each person has a task. The management of patients seems regulated in an optimal way. Their level of hygiene is impressive. Such cleanliness, such neatness, implies a meticulous and systematic organization. I imagine the population's general education contributes as well. How else to explain that, despite all the patients coming and going, the care unit stays so immaculate? Undoubtedly, American children are taught rules, manners, and respect. There is a terrible lack of that in the countries I know, such as the Tibet of my childhood, where an outdated lifestyle carries on today, but also in China, Nepal, and India. At one point, I was admitted to a well-managed Chinese military hospital, but it was only a pale imitation of this emergency ward. I leave Bellevue admiring and confident. I am reassured. The American doctors will certainly find the solution to avoid recurrences on my right foot, and they will heal the disease that has been gnawing my ankle since my arrest. I thank Jigme and make him promise that the next time we will make sure Rigzin Dolma is there.

The treatment I am given is effective; my pain eases while I am still in the emergency ward. Going back to Thinley's seems shorter and less painful. My optimism, however, is soon destroyed by a new fit of violent pain, even more violent than the previous ones. The purple skin breaks on my very swollen ankle and becomes an open, foul-smelling wound. I wrap it in toilet paper, covering it as best I can with a sock. I decide not to wait the prescribed two weeks. This time, I make an appointment with Rigzin Dolma for a consultation.

The Program for Survivors of Torture

On May 23, 2003, Rigzin Dolma is waiting for me in the entrance hall of Bellevue, and I follow her into her office. With a few clicks on her computer, my name — which I am still unable to write in English — appears on the screen. I have a medical record, with an identification number, which was created when I first came to the emergency ward. I am not unknown anymore.

I can see immediately that the doctor examining me is worried about my case. After a lengthy examination and palpation of my leg, he sends me to radiology. I am ashamed of my foot and of its smell. I feel like asking questions that Dolma could translate, but I do not dare. A nurse brings in a wheelchair, and Dolma accompanies me through a maze of sanitized corridors. Once in the waiting room of the radiology department, she tells me her story. Through her, I discover the Tibetans of the diaspora whom I have never had the chance to meet before. It amuses me to hear her speaking Tibetan with no accent but with American expressions and body language. She expresses herself quite openly, and she easily confides straightaway in a stranger. It is unlike the culture of secrecy that prevails in Tibet, even among close relations, even within families.

This twenty-seven-year-old woman, born in New York City, belongs to the second generation of exiles. Her parents grew up on the Nepalese slope of Mount Everest, in Jyalsa, in the Sherpa area of Solukhumbu. When Nepal, under pressure from the Chinese, tightened its policy on Tibetan refugees, her family jumped at the opportunity to emigrate to the United States in 1970. Dolma remembers her father's pride when, as soon as she had learned to read, he had her decipher his family name in the New York City directory. Her mother, Choeden, was the youngest in a family of fifteen children; as a child, she was in charge of preparing the offerings of water and light in the morning. She enjoyed honoring the Buddha in that way, but she regretted not having bowls and finely plated lamps like the ones she admired in temples. Therefore, she is happy today that, in the back of a photocopy store in Queens, she has a table of ritual objects and handicrafts that she sells to local Tibetans.

Dolma is a certified nurse, and she has been engaged to Tenzin Nyima for two years. She is proud to tell me about this young man, who is the assistant manager of the organization Students for a Free Tibet, which is a worldwide network supporting the Tibetan cause. He grew up in the Tibetan Children's Village in Dharamsala, India. He speaks Tibetan, English, Hindi, and Chinese perfectly well. As a former Fulbright Scholar, he has a degree in law and international relations from Harvard University. After being a consultant at the National Endowment for Democracy* in Washington, DC, he moved to New York City, and they met during a March 10 demonstration commemorating the anniversary of the 1959 Tibetan Uprising.

We are interrupted by the radiographer, who takes several X-rays of my foot, my right leg, my lungs, and my spine. After that, Dolma leads me to the laboratory for a blood test. Finally, we see the doctor about these tests. He first speaks with Dolma for a few minutes. Not being able to understand grieves me. My inability to communicate makes me feel not fully human. Without language, I feel like an animal.

Dolma's face seems clouded. She explains to me that I am suffering from an infectious disease that requires my hospitalization. But I can sense that she is holding back information. The hospital's administration needs me to give details on my incarceration in Tibet so that I can be accepted in the Program for Survivors of Torture. The doctor suggests that I be hospitalized immediately for observation. In front of the doctor, I do not question Dolma, and I am rather relieved to be granted this providential treatment, thus avoiding having to go back to Thinley's flat.

I am taken to a spacious room whose whiteness delights me. I have never enjoyed such comfort. I do not link illness to such luxury. There is no doubt in my mind that, in such an environment, the chances are I will soon be cured. Dolma informs me that an American interpreter will come visit me. She speaks Tibetan fluently, and she will attend me during consultations and for the administrative procedures. The young woman seems uncomfortable, and I do not want to bother her any longer by forcing her

---

* The National Endowment for Democracy (NED) is a private, nonprofit foundation dedicated to the growth and strengthening of democratic institutions around the world; it is largely funded by the U.S. Congress.

to tell me what she is concealing. For the moment, I am entirely absorbed in the pleasure of my unexpected living conditions and filled with gratitude for this country, where penniless foreigners are taken care of free of charge. In Tibet, China, Nepal, or India, people die every day because they are not granted access to a hospital. Though I have hardly arrived in the United States, I am benefiting from such generosity!

I cannot believe it. Just then, a nurse knocks on the door, and she comes in with a smile and supper on a tray. I am staggered, embarrassed by such thoughtfulness. She hands me a glass of water, and using signs, she asks me to swallow four capsules. They are probably analgesics, for I am suffering much less. The bed is soft, and the smooth sheets smell nice and fresh. I cannot believe I am lying on such a firm and thick mattress. The bed's control system allows me to raise my head or my feet to the exact desired height. As I delight in these facilities, I pray that I might some day in my life allow other sick people to enjoy such comfort. How can I not remember the bed and the room I occupied when I first arrived at Sera Mey Monastery in the south of India?

It was in 1985, and it was difficult for Tibetan monks to survive in exile. Communities were constantly expanding due to the continuous influx of newcomers who were leaving Tibet to come to India to study the Dharma, which was banished in our native country. There were four of us in a tiny room, and our beds were in fact layers of stems and stalks of dry corn. We would pick the stalks up in the dump of a neighboring village, for they were too rough and too knotty for fodder. Then we would pile them up within a rectangular frame of four more-or-less-fitted wooden planks, with a shawl on top. The fabric was very thin, as we did not have the means to treat ourselves to a thicker one. The bumps of the stems and stalks of corn tore the fabric very quickly. Our skin was not spared. In the morning, our bodies were marked with the shapes of the ears and stalks, and we were sometimes bruised and scratched if we had slept too long in the same position. Worse yet, all kinds of insects — such as weevils, bugs, spiders, ring-worms, fleas, lice, and other sorts of vermin — would come to suck our blood during the night! When we shook out our shawls in the morning, we could see them trailing away in black processions, but we knew they would be back that evening.

As a young monk, I dreamed of owning a mattress. I found out the price, and I worked out what I could save on the meager donations I received during rituals. Day after day, I set aside the number of rupees I needed. At last, I was indeed able to buy myself a mattress...but of very mediocre comfort! In the hospital, I am overwhelmed by the strangeness of my fate! I had to become ill, and disabled, and travel over six thousand miles from my birthplace to be able at last to sleep in a real bed! My masters taught me, when I started my studies, that suffering purifies. In this moment, my conclusion is that the terrible pain of these past weeks has washed the bad karma that has, until now, not allowed me to sleep comfortably.

CHAPTER FIVE

Cutting Is Not Curing:
I Refuse Amputation

Marina Illich Looks Like Her Country

"What exactly have you been told about your illness?"

Seated at my bedside in my hospital room, a young American woman with an expressive face is speaking perfect Tibetan from Lhasa. Marina Illich is a PhD student from Columbia University who studies under Professor Robert Thurman. She is writing a thesis on Changkya Rölpé Dorjé, a remarkable lama who lived in the eighteenth century. Respected for the depth of his spiritual achievement, and for his understanding of the scriptures, he was also the mentor and the consultant of Emperor Qianlong in Peking, to whom he skillfully defended the interests of Tibet. At the time, the emperor — called the Son of Heaven — would prostrate himself with devotion before the master of the Potala — the Dalai Lama — whom he worshipped as a living Buddha and his spiritual refuge. In the name of the sacred links of *chod-yon* — "Protective Guru" — the Sino-Manchurian court of the Qin officially recognized the Dalai Lama as the political and religious sovereign of the Land of Snow, defending it against the forays of the fearsome Mongolian armies, as well as against the internal unrest caused by rivalries between Tibetan warlords.

I assess Marina's scholarship as, filled with admiration, she tells me about her professor, Robert Thurman. If there are two Americans that all diaspora Tibetans know, they are undoubtedly Robert Thurman and the actor Richard Gere. Bob — as we call him in the nicely unaffected way that is so common among people in the United States — was the first Westerner to be ordained a monk by the Dalai Lama. A brilliant scholar, and the son of a United Nations interpreter, he radically gave up his golden but superficial life. Fascinated by meditation and Buddhist philosophy, he made a trip in 1962 to Dharamsala and became the Dalai Lama's friend. To better understand Buddhist scriptures, he learned Tibetan, and in 1964, he was ordained a monk at Namgyal, Kundun's private monastery. Life called him back to the United States, and three years later, in 1967, he resigned his vows in order to marry a dazzlingly beautiful Swedish aristocrat, who was also a top model and a psychotherapist. Later, Bob created the Je Tsongkhapa chair of Tibetan Studies at Columbia University — where he is teaching when I meet Marina — and at the request of the Dalai Lama, he founded — along with Richard Gere — Tibet House, which fights against the cultural genocide in Tibet. Robert Thurman has rallied several members of the U.S. Senate to defend human rights in Tibet, and he has contributed to the international influence of the Mind & Life Institute's symposiums, which began as dialogues between the Dalai Lama and leading scientists on the mind and the self. One day, the Dalai Lama paid tribute to Bob's life, which has been dedicated to teaching the Dharma and to human values, by fondly stating with some humor that it will be necessary to go in search of his reincarnation when he leaves his body! The next generation would then see the reappearance of a Bob Rinpoche!

I recall all this as Marina sits in front of me. I also notice that the wind of karma is confronting me with a terrible ordeal, all while sending the right persons to my bedside to help me go through it. Lost in my thoughts, I answer noncommittally. Marina can see how difficult it is for me to confide in her, but she is not the kind of woman to give up. She insists. When she realizes that I know very little about my illness, she falls silent. I can see she has some bad news to give me — the something that Dolma did not want to tell me yesterday.

She pulls the medical report out of her bag. To understand it, not only do I need a Tibetan translation but also a textual analysis. We engage in a word-for-word translation that objectivizes the symptoms I have been suffering since January 2000: "There is generalized osteopenia. There is marked bone resorption and fragmentation at the ankle joint, involving the tibial plafond and talar dome suspicious for septic arthritis. The tarsal bones are not well visualized, and appear largely fused. Findings suspicious for septic arthritis of the ankle joint; fusion of the intertarsal joints noted."

This is the first time I hear the medical terms *osteopenia* and *arthritis*, which are absolutely unpronounceable for me. Marina endeavors to explain them. Osteopenia means a severe loss of bone density, while arthritis is an acute or chronic inflammation of the joints. Arthritis often affects athletes because they endlessly repeat the same movements using the same joints. In my case, the origin is traumatic, and Marina asks me to confirm that my problems were really caused by police brutality.

At this point, I am not worried. I even reassure Marina: "It's an incredible chance for me to have been admitted in this hospital. In India, there would be no way for me to be taken care of, but here, I will inevitably be cured."

Confronted by her doubtful look, I add: "Even if it takes time…"

She answers that I will undoubtedly heal, but that it will not be easy. The process might take a long time, it might be painful, and there is a serious risk that I might lose my right leg. Seeing my X-ray, the doctor who examined me does not rule out amputation below my knee.

"But it's only Dr. Jones's opinion," she immediately explains. "For such serious cases, it is always necessary to consult other specialists."

She is surprised when I say: "If amputation is the solution, it is not a problem! American surgeons do that very well, don't they?"

Marina approves. However, since all we have is a first report, she advises me to wait and see how things develop with the treatment, and she explains in detail the medicines I have to take and for what reason. Antibiotics, anti-inflammatories — my vocabulary is becoming richer. At the thought of becoming an expert in medical terminology, I smile and remain deeply optimistic. I joke and point out to Marina that I feel more confident about the American care system than she does. She agrees and asks me to get psychologically prepared for the interview I will need to go through to be accepted in the Program for Survivors of Torture. I will have to tell about my arrest, my incarceration, and the physical abuse I underwent. Admittedly, this is not easy, but I am aware that I cannot shirk this protocol. I agree and try to relax Marina.

Her concern does not wear down my good mood. I am infinitely grateful to Tara, my guardian, for having put this attentive and devoted young American woman on my path. We talk for almost two hours. Marina Illich looks like her country, which I have been getting to know for three weeks. Energetic, willful, determined, persistent, and undoubtedly a perfectionist, she also has a brilliant mind. Yet I can sense that she seeks more than new challenges and intellectual achievements. She serves a code of ethics and humanity. Though I cannot assess its depth, I can feel it and I am delighted for her. I admire her intellectual capacities.

It is so difficult for me to utter a few words of English, or to remember the names of the doctors I consult, while she speaks impeccable Tibetan, which she took only four years to learn without ever having been to Tibet. She has also studied Chinese and speaks Hungarian — since her father comes from Budapest — and French, as she was born in Brussels and lived there for the first few years of her life. Marina joined the Program for Survivors of Torture as a volunteer translator for medical consultations. The program often welcomes former Tibetan political prisoners and is always in need of interpreters, so a program manager wrote to Professor Robert Thurman, who made an announcement to his students. As it happened, Marina was already interested in Tibetan spirituality, and she kept herself informed of news regarding the deprivation of human rights and fundamental freedom in Tibet.

I Am Suffering from Gangrene

On June 4, Marina goes with me to see the orthopedic surgeon. We have had several conversations, and I continue to believe that, if amputation is the necessary solution, I will consider it without hesitation. Dr. Ali, who is of Pakistani origin, greets us, with his datebook lying open before him. He has been given my X-rays, and without any preliminaries, he describes the protocol awaiting me. I will continue the antibiotic therapy I am already following, and I will see a physiotherapist for two months in order to make the muscles of my right thigh stronger to compensate for the loss of my right leg below the knee. Given this timeframe, he suggests scheduling the operation for the week of August 4. As he is in the operating room on Tuesdays, Thursdays, and Fridays, Dr. Ali suggests amputating my leg on the morning of Thursday, August 7.

I am surprised at his abruptness, which contrasts sharply with the affability I have experienced until now. I do not say a word. The surgeon shows me the prosthesis that I will be fitted with once the wound is healed. I joke that though I now have the leg of an elephant, after the operation it will be the leg of a mouse. I say, "Too bad! I would have preferred to remain a lama with an elephant leg!"

Marina smiles, but Dr. Ali remains impassive. He turns his computer screen toward me and shows me a video of amputated people who not only can walk but can run, jump, climb stairs, dance, swim, climb mountains, ski, ride a bicycle, and parachute from airplanes....I have never done that much!

Oddly, upon seeing these pictures, I feel increasingly reluctant to accept amputation, though I had accepted it at first. Maybe it's because I am discovering its reality, but I am unsure. I just hear an inner voice whispering to me: *Don't accept amputation! Don't accept amputation!*

The surgeon finishes his demonstration. He gives me an appointment for three weeks later. Till then, I must submit to a series of medical exams, and I have to meet the physiotherapist in charge of preparing me. As Dr. Ali writes down his name, I emerge from my silence. I share my doubts with Marina. She understands my confusion and is shocked herself by the course of this conversation. The doctor has mostly soliloquized for three-quarters of an hour without paying any attention to me. She tells the doctor that I need to think about it.

Dr. Ali does not budge. Marina adds: "It is a difficult decision to make. We have planned to see other specialists. We will come back to you."

The surgeon lifts his eyes and frowns, looking sternly from under his thick and heavy black eyebrows. He speaks to us as if we are scatterbrains who don't understand the consequences of our choices: "I cannot save the date of August 7 indefinitely. Don't take too long informing me of your decision. The X-rays are positive. I would be surprised if you were not advised amputation. And you must understand that gangrene cannot wait. If you are not operated on quickly, it is not below the knee that your leg will have to be cut, but below your hip. After that, I will accept no responsibility. Gangrene is lethal."

Marina turns pale. The doctor does not wait for her to translate his speech for me. He gets up, gives us a cold nod, and sits back down behind his desk as we make our way out.

We stop at a vending machine. Marina sips a fruit juice, trying to relax, but she cannot calm her indignation. Dr. Ali has not spared us.

"I understand your not wanting to follow up," she says. "I would have done the same, and if there is no other solution than amputation, let's find another surgeon!"

She offers to call a cousin, a renowned orthopedic surgeon, who operates in a private clinic on the banks of the Hudson River. I think this is a good idea. Rather than getting in a panic after this morning's consultation, we should take time to reflect. This is only a setback, probably caused by a lack of communication. Perhaps Dr. Ali has only recently arrived in the United States and has not yet acquired the good manners of Americans.

"Let it go, Rinpoche. We'll find a way," quips Marina, whose smile reappears as she pushes my wheelchair.

I sense that something else is bothering her, and upon arriv-ing in my room, I urge her to tell me everything quite frankly. What awaits me is not easy, and on this presumably long path, we must be as open as possible with one another.

"The doctor said a word that worries me," Marina tells me. "I don't understand because I did not see it in the X-ray report. But it is maybe a word for the general public. The radiologist spoke of septic arthritis, and Dr. Ali mentioned gangrene."

Gangrene? This new word will quickly become familiar. Afraid of demoralizing me, Marina explains that gangrene is a process in which cells die because they cannot regenerate due to a lack of blood circulation. In my case, for example, because of an infection. Deprived of oxygen, tissues can rot very quickly. They blacken and start weeping.

I say, "So it is just a question of reactivating blood circulation? That shouldn't be too complicated?"

Neophyte that I am, I think American medicine should be able to deal with such a problem. It solves much worse cases. How can medical professionals who perform open-heart surgeries and succeed in transplanting hearts and kidneys not overcome a foot infection? I reassure Marina and try to convince her that, in spite of appearances, it was very good to meet this Pakistani doctor this morning. It's good he mentioned gangrene. At least now I understand what illness I am suffering from. I am relieved to know that, to heal, my blood needs to circulate correctly down to my foot again. I have not the slightest doubt that this can be done.

Marina smiles at my optimism, which nothing seems to abate. She promises to call her cousin and to return quickly with news. I thank her for all the time she is giving me and for her efforts to help me understand my illness.

Cutting Is Not Curing!

Every morning, a nurse comes to cleanse my wound. It is the most painful moment of the day. The painkillers have yet to provide any relief when the nurse inserts into my purulent ankle a metallic instrument in the shape of a tiny spoon, a curette. Its tip and its edges are as sharp as a razor blade, and I am astonished to see that the instrument goes right into my ankle with no difficulty. I realize that the joint is so ravaged by gangrene that it is hollowed out to the point of being empty. I ask Marina to explain the reason for this treatment. The goal, she says, is to open the wound so that, hopefully, buds of healthy skin might pass along some specialized repairing cells into the gangrenous tissue. These cells have the ability to clean areas with necrosis and to regenerate immunity by producing the appropriate antibodies.

Understanding that helps me accept this aggressive treatment. My open wounds now ooze with blood, but this is in order to allow the regrowth of new healthy tissues and ultimately to heal. Added to the pain, there is the foul smell, which is, I am told, distinctive of insufficiently irrigated tissues. Anaerobic bacteria, which causes flesh to decay, proliferates in the wound, along with purulent secretions.

The curetting takes about twenty minutes. This amounts to one-third of an hour, and if that is the price to pay for a natural process of healing, I would accept a second session! But I am told that the repair cells need at least twenty-four hours to work.

On June 12, I have an appointment with Dr. Jones, who prescribed me the antibiotics. He is fortyish, a very gentle and smiling man. There is great peacefulness and a marked benevolence in the way he looks, speaks, and listens. My right ankle shows no sign of improvement, and the pus secretions have worsened despite the daily curetting. Dr. Jones concludes I have a severe infection in my bones, and my leg will need to be amputated.

If my wound has not changed, I, on the other hand, have changed. Confronted with this diagnosis, and with more advice to amputate immediately, I ask Marina to explain to the doctor that, in my mind, I believe I can cure. I only need help in restoring blood circulation in my ankle. I beg the doctor to prescribe medication aiming at that. He sighs. Now that I have reached this stage — aside from curetting and taking more antibiotics, which have not yielded any results — he can offer no other solution than amputation.

I reply that improvement of my health will certainly take time, but that I am willing to be patient. Dr. Jones warns me that waiting to operate risks letting the infection spread to the upper part of my leg and becoming widespread.

"Come back in two months," he says in conclusion, and he extends my prescription of antibiotics.

Three days later, Marina introduces me to her cousin Arnold, the surgeon. His elegant apartment, filled with lacquered, sepia furniture, is located on the Upper West Side. From its large plate-glass windows, I gaze at the Manhattan skyline. Aglow at sundown, it seems so fragile, so vulnerable! It is hard for me to believe that it's a real metropolis with millions of inhabitants! As the evening settles in, the skyscrapers become an immaterial screen of luminous cubes. Their edges form well-designed and clear-cut threads, perpendicular to the streets and squared out with shafts of light. In this cityscape of glass and concrete, such brilliance, such perfection, verges on unreality. I seem to be gazing at the gigantic setting of some megalomaniacal delusion laid down on the banks of the Hudson River. The peaceful waters form a dark green corridor. Sidelong beams fall into it, going from one street to the next between the buildings. They mark out an angle of incidental light on the river's surface, like blades cutting through the water, stabbing the Hudson.

Arnold examines me carefully and looks at the X-ray of my foot for a long time. He turns to Marina, and though I'm not able to understand English, I can guess that he is confirming the conclusions made by the other doctors. He sounds positive, with no room for doubt. Besides, I now recognize these two final words: *gangrene* and *amputation*. Even before Marina translates, I tell her, with the new-forged determination I have acquired during my three weeks of hospitalization: "I do not want to have my leg cut! I want it to be cured!"

For more than an hour, as Marina translates, Arnold justifies amputation. No matter how often I repeat "Cutting is not curing!" the doctor continues to insist that my foot is dead. The necrosis has gone too far; the ankle joint absolutely cannot recover. The bones and the cartilage are destroyed. Arnold speaks highly of prosthesis. He offers to show me the same video as Dr. Ali, but I have already seen it and it has not convinced me.

"Rinpoche prefers being a lama with an elephant leg rather than with the leg of a mouse," Marina jokes, repeating my expression.

I do my best to hide my disappointment. I was expecting a lot from this consultation. I share my confusion with Marina. Why don't the doctors I meet suggest anything other than cutting my leg? How can a civilization that sends men to the moon not know how to cure a gangrenous leg?

Marina, who is also puzzled, has already reflected on these questions. She is the niece of Ivan Illich, a unique thinker, visionary essayist, and controversial social critic. Illich died in December 2002, less than a year ago, and the two of them had been very close.

Marina was fascinated by her uncle and his critiques of the dysfunctions of postindustrial society. For instance, Ivan Illich proposed that the level of sophistication reached in the richest countries had become counterproductive. Citing the alienation and illusions the Western care system caused in people, he claimed that doctors sometimes cured illness in ways that were detrimental to the patient's health. I was just beginning to understand this personally. Cutting a leg is relatively easy when you have the sophisticated technical ability to do so. But how could doctors reduce the art of curing to plain and simple amputation without even attempting to treat me in other ways? Why did they have the nerve to assert that my ankle was dead?

I am shocked to uncover this reality. I begin to see that I have been deluding myself by believing that the political, economic, and military omnipotence of the United States would also apply to its health care. I came to New York City convinced that the ailment of my foot would be cured, and I have maintained that illusion since my admission at Bellevue. I am becoming disenchanted.

Moreover, Marina adds that her uncle was so convinced that patients die of curing at the hands of doctors that he never accepted treatment for the cancerous tumor in his right jaw. Rather than be operated on, he let the tumor slowly deform his face during the last twenty years of his life. Even when it came to his own health, he remained consistent, matching his actions with his thoughts. In fact, he considered cancers to be the typical example of illnesses that are treated in a counterproductive way. Surgery might have ruined his ability to speak, which he could not abide, and he was convinced he would have died sooner had he allowed the operation.

Marina opens my eyes with her uncle's example. As for my case, the cause of the problem has been identified: It is the absence of life-bearing oxygen in my ankle. There must be a doctor who is able to outline an appropriate medical protocol.

"It seems simple when you say that," remarks Marina. "But the problem is that all the doctors that we have consulted until now, Arnold included, all of them say that your ankle is dead."

I challenge this point. No, my ankle is not dead, I tell her. It is giving all the signs of irreversible necrosis on the X-rays of the radiologists, but I have a precise sensation telling me deep down inside that there is still life in it, despite the septic arthritis — or whatever the name of my illness. Though life in my ankle is weakened, faint, meager to the point of not being detected with X-rays, it is still alive.

The Liberating Strength of Forgiveness

Two days later, overcome with doubt, with my chances of healing lessening, I have to revisit my past. The date of the interview for the admission procedure at Bellevue Hospital arrives. I have been preparing for it with Marina, whose presence at my side is a great comfort. How to tell my story? How can I translate into words the horrors I experienced in prison?

My story is altogether unusual and very commonplace. It is commonplace among those in the Tibetan diaspora. The eleven refugees sharing Thinley's apartment have all been through incarceration, torture, and physical abuse. But these are silent sufferings. How can one talk about them? How can one share them with those who have not experienced "hell on Earth" in the Chinese People's Republic jails? Americans enjoy the respect of human rights in their country so much that they do not always understand how precious these rights are and how much they have to be defended.

"Our Constitution," explains Marina, "is based on liberty, equality, *and* happiness. We tend to forget that, in a moral sense, *happiness* means it is our duty to make others around us happy, not only to seek selfish satisfaction of our desires. Our democracy has been, since its origin, founded on the idea of happiness. In another value system, what might appear as social injustice is considered in the United States as a moral transgression. For, in the logic of American democracy, happiness must remain the mission inscribed in our Constitution by the Founding Fathers, as a right and a civic duty."

Throughout my years of exile in the West, I have realized that democracy does not mean sharing the riches, but I have noticed that it ensures the protection of each person and everyone. For me, having suffered deprivation of fundamental liberties, this is of capital importance. Furthermore, the American social agreement is that individuals are promised that society will open up for them, without being hindered by their origins. Americans all share the same dream, and the most destitute knows that one's circumstances are not inevitable. Tomorrow, one can become rich and powerful. But at the time, I am so overcome by the shock of such a radically different environment that I am completely disoriented. Everything is new: the lifestyle, the ways of communicating and thinking, the behaviors, the language. Thanks to Marina, I am given the essential keys to decipher this world, but I am far from having found my bearings.

The interview with the psychologist for my admission in the Program for Survivors of Torture will last two hours. I know these two hours will stir up many sufferings — first of all, my present condition as a refugee. I have been greeted with tremendous generosity at Bellevue Hospital. But, at this point, I have lost everything, including my health. The interview will also bring back the shameful denial of humanity that I was subjected to in Chinese jails. Not being human any longer, being reduced to the despicable dregs of society, with a dismantled body, dismembered by torture, humiliated by degrading treatments — how can I express all of this to human beings whose physical and moral integrity have never been trampled? It will feel as if I am attacking their intact humanity by displaying my own violated humanity.

I have never told anyone about my experience in prison, neither people close to me nor my masters. When I met the Dalai Lama after my escape, I did not need to describe to him my tortures. He knows only too well what goes on in the prisons of the Roof of the World. Without asking me any questions, he hugged me silently. Then he simply said: "Three months of prison and torture! It's a terrible ordeal! But for others, it lasts ten years, twenty years! It kills some!"

I understood then how important it is to put our sufferings into perspective, to not lock oneself in a painful past that indefinitely extends the ordeal. When that happens, we become our own torturer.

On June 17, 2003, in the office of the Program for Survivors of Torture, I am greeted by the psychologist, a smiling young woman with the blue eyes of a doll. Her manners are demonstrative, and her kindness is conventional, both features of social relations in the United States. I have not yet gotten used to this in the weeks that have gone by, and I must seem very coarse to some of the people I speak with. Indeed, my culture is not very exuberant.

Although I can see this young woman intends to be genuinely benevolent and open to my story, a misunderstanding quickly arises between us as soon as I mention my detention and tortures. I will soon realize that Westerners easily indulge in victimization. This explains their amazement, and their total lack of understanding, when I joke about the ill treatments I suffered in prison.

In her eventual report, the Bellevue psychologist will state: "Mr. Dorje's affect was stable, however, it seemed inappropriate at times. For example, he was smiling, animated, and even laughed as he described his torture in detail, and his survival."

She would have better understood my feelings had I acted like a punching bag and expressed myself with the tearful language of complaint. Then she would have sympathized and undoubtedly shared my wailing, my indignation, my anger, and my hatred toward my torturers. During our interview, I got the impression that she was driving me into a corner and wanting me to accuse my tormentors. That was when I burst out laughing.

How can I take on a hatred I do not feel?

In fact, on that day, even if I was only a penniless refugee, and a sick man with a gangrenous leg, I was not the victim. The victims were my jailers. I had left prison, but what about them? They were locked up in a vicious spiral that would hound them during this life and for many lives yet to come!

The psychologist did not understand that I laughed at the absurdity of hating those who had shown such hatred toward me. During my incarceration, I was often dumbfounded at the idea that people who did not know me, and whom I had never been harmful to, could relentlessly torture me. And I have meditated at length on karmic causality. What was happening to me was only the result, the consequence, of a negative spirit and negative thoughts that, in previous lives, had led me to injure and cause pain to other beings, human and nonhuman. My torturers were not my enemies. The real enemy is not outside of us. It is to be confronted within us. It takes the shape of selfishness, attachment, self-cherishing. I was therefore laughing at how absurd hatred, thirst for revenge, and anger are. By laughing, I was hoping to relax Marina and the psychologist. But I only managed to make them tense.

Sometimes, when I think of the bad karma built up by the People's Armed Police officers who tortured me, I feel tremendous compassion for them. Moved to tears, I pray for them more than for anyone else. And I have completely forgiven them. It is only thanks to my forgiveness that one day, as soon as possible I hope, they may free themselves from their infernal karma.

In appearance they were the torturers and I the victim. But in reality, we were all victims. I was their physical punching bag, and they were the victims of their own uncontrollable, destructive emotions. For lack of purifying the actions they committed to ensure the meager sustenance of their families, they will experience the terrible torments of being reborn as hungry ghosts, hot or cold hellish beings, or animals.... How can I know? I dedicate to them the positive energy of my praiseworthy actions so that they may find peace of mind at last.

Talking to the psychologist at Bellevue Hospital, how can I explain that the understanding of karma I developed in prison freed me from the unbearable burden of negative emotions? I thus feel gratitude toward those who tortured me. They taught me patience, unconditional compassion, and impartiality, more than any of my masters have. Every day, I express my wishes for them, and offer them my prayers, so that they may free themselves from mental states upset by hatred and anger. Has the psychologist in front of me ever heard about karma? I doubt that it was part of her studies. If it had been, she would express herself differently.

The law of karma implies that we must assume our share of responsibility in what happens to us. This is easier in the case of happiness and when positive developments occur in our life. But in adversity, I find this a source of deep wisdom. It has allowed me to become friends with what I would otherwise deem bad and therefore reject. As it is said in one of the fundamental teachings I meditated on during my training at the monastery:

> When the container and the contents are full of negativity,
> Transform adverse fortune into an Awakening path.
> Use all immediate circumstances in meditation.

I have therefore fully accepted the idea that I created the causes of my detention through actions whose essence came to maturity in this life, and I am delighted at having cleansed these negativities. Such an attitude has transformed the way I see those who brutalized me with unimaginable barbarity. Through the sufferings they inflicted on me, they created the necessary conditions for my transformation. How can I not feel infinitely grateful to them?

Aware of the subtleties of karmic causality, while electric

baton blows were showering on me, I meditated, body and soul, on these verses by the great Tibetan saint Langri Tangpa:*

> When I see beings of unpleasant character,
> Oppressed by strong negativity and suffering,
> May I hold them dear — for they are rare to find —
> As if I have discovered a jewel treasure!

My Arrest

In the interview, the psychologist feels ill at ease when I express compassion for those who tortured me, so she asks me to describe the reasons for, and the conditions of, my arrest. She is disconcerted when I tell her it was another life. I try to be as factual as possible and only share the minimum information that is necessary to be admitted in the Program for Survivors of Torture.

It is spring 1997, seventy-five hundred miles away from New York City. I am thirty-one years old. At the request of the Dalai Lama, I have returned to Ashi Monastery, near Lithang, where I have been enthroned as the abbot. I teach the monks, and the lay population, the basic principles of Buddhism, which they do not necessarily put into practice and have partly forgotten after forty years of communist indoctrination. Compassion is one of the most precious jewels of our culture, the heart of Illumination. In *The Way of the Bodhisattva*, the great saint Shantideva praises the great compassion that has neither limit nor bias:

> This is the supreme draft of immortality
> That slays the Lord of Death, the slaughterer of beings,
> The rich unfailing treasure-mine
> To heal the poverty of wanderers.

---

* Geshe Langri Tangpa (1054–1123) is famous throughout Tibet for his "Eight Verses of Training the Mind," which have been the subject of numerous commentaries, and he is revered as an emanation of Amitabha Buddha.

It is the sovereign remedy
That perfectly allays all maladies.
It is the tree that gives relief
To those who wander wearily the pathways of existence.
It is the universal bridge that saves
All wandering beings from the states of loss,
The rising moon of the enlightened mind
That soothes the sorrows born of afflictions.
It is the mighty sun that utterly dispels
The misty ignorance of wandering beings,
The creamy butter, rich and full,
That's churned from milk of holy teaching.

It is my duty to introduce the essence of compassion as well as how to implement it in everyday life. Therefore, I advise the inhabitants not to follow the Chinese custom of excessively hunting deer to the point where the species might be endangered. That will be a first charge against me.

The Dharma is a teaching that frees the mind from basic ignorance, which is at the root of suffering. I speak about the final freedom born from wisdom, when the mind recognizes its true loving, and radiant, nature. Mentioning freedom will be a second charge against me.

Finally, as is the custom, I have placed on the main throne in Ashi a big portrait of His Holiness the Dalai Lama, the incarnation on Earth of Awakened Compassion. That will be a third charge against me.

In November 1998, I am found guilty of actions aimed at destabilizing the motherland. The officer who questions me, from the Chinese People's Armed Police Force, has piercing, constantly moving eyes. His chubby face reminds me of a marmot about to hibernate. In contrast with his appearance, which could seem good-natured, he speaks curtly, his voice rising to an unnaturally

high pitch. He orders me not to speak about freedom, neither publicly nor privately, and not to say anything anymore that would
seem antigovernmental to the lay population. He also requires me
to denounce the Dalai Lama. These demands are consistent with
the police force's "Strike Hard" campaign, which uses the slogan
"Strike hard and eliminate separatists!" I will quickly discover that,
without knowing it, and despite myself, I am a separatist.

The Chinese have recently held a series of official meetings
in Lhasa, in which they have reaffirmed the need to intensify the
hard-line policy. They focus on repressing religious institutions,
the "hotbeds of dissidence." Their goal is to eradicate the internal
and secret separatist groups, in particular former exiles, like me,
who have come back to the country. The People's Armed Police
suspects us of being linked with the so-called "Dalai's clique,"
which is a decided fantasy of die-hard proponents of the Cultural
Revolution. The main strategies of the authorities are patriotic
reeducation, which targets monasteries and convents, and drastic
security measures to prevent the infiltration of antigovernment
documents, such as photographs of the Dalai Lama, recordings of
his teachings, and Dharma books. Being in possession of any of
these amounts to a crime against state security, which could earn
a sentence of several years of hard labor.

Many neighboring monasteries have been ransacked by the
army, and several lamas have been arrested. I understand, at the
end of my summons, that sooner or later it will be my turn. Two
months later, on January 28, 1999, at 11 PM, the police come to
arrest me. They first take me to the Public Security office, where
I am bound hand and foot. Then they throw a cloth bag over my
head and shovel me into the trailer of a car that roars off. We
drive through the night, and at one point, the vehicle turns onto
a mud track and slows down. The guards throw me overboard. I
get back up, one eyebrow cut, my head covered with blood, and I

stagger a few steps in the dark. I then slip into a muddy rut and am unable to catch myself, since my hands are tied. I twist my right foot and crash down onto the ground again, face to the earth. My nose starts bleeding a lot. Soldiers arrive and give me a volley of blows from head to foot and into the stomach. They pull me up and order me to walk. I try to make my way despite my right leg, which cannot carry me anymore, and despite my dizziness. As I proceed slowly, the soldiers shower blows onto me even more. I am thrown, unconscious, onto the icy concrete floor of a cell.

Incarceration and Escape

Thus, the hardest three months of my life begin. The authorities of the detention center want me to confess that I correspond regularly, in secret, with the Dalai Lama, therefore putting state security in danger. The questionings are carried out daily by Chinese or Tibetan officers of the People's Armed Police, from 10 AM until early afternoon. They last about a week, and then they are interrupted after five or six days. The goal of the tortures I regularly undergo is to make me confess. The confession will then be presented at court, where I will be sentenced. Considering the charges against me, I risk twenty years of reeducation through work, maybe even life imprisonment. But I deny outright all accusations of separatism. I am not a spy in the pay of the Dalai Lama, trained in the Tibetan diaspora of India. My only mission in life is to teach the Dharma, in the service of those who suffer.

In prison, food and drink are very insufficient: only a piece of bread and raw potato soup, morning and evening. In such conditions, my health deteriorates quickly. The wound on my feet worsening, I try to be hospitalized. It is not easy, for even injured prisoners are not granted medical treatment, or they are treated too late. Those who survive often have permanent disabilities. I remember the case of a young nun who had spent three years in prison with a broken arm, which she suffered during her arrest in Lhasa in the spring of 1993. Her arm was broken by the butt of a gun, and the wound was never cured; it even got worse because she was forced to do the cleaning and the gardening. After her liberation, she was crippled for life, since her flesh had grown around the broken bone.

At the end of March 1999, thanks to my insistence, I am escorted by two policemen and admitted into a military hospital. I receive good medical treatment, and my ankle is operated on. The surgeon lances lateral incisions on the right and left sides. I recover quickly. Yet I know that, upon full recovery, I will have to go back to prison. I will be tortured again, then tried and heavily sentenced. So I try to strategize a way to escape, as soon as my foot is strong enough.

The guard on duty in front of my room inevitably takes a nap after his lunch. He sleeps so soundly that, from my bed, I can hear him snoring. I make arrangements to find civilian clothes, and one afternoon in July 1999, I put them on. Taking advantage of the sleeping guard, I leave my room — the door of which is not locked. Fortunately, I am at the end of a corridor, near service stairs. I go downstairs without meeting anyone. The last risk is if someone from the nursing team recognizes me in the entrance hall. I walk with my head lowered, a cap pulled over my forehead, and step over the threshold without mishap. I then take a bus to Lhasa, where I live as a recluse for almost one year. So it is that, in April 2000, I attempt to cross the Himalayas to Nepal and India, to freedom.

In Bellevue Hospital, it is the first time I tell the story of this journey. It boils down to a two-hour conversation and a three-page report, written by the psychologist of the Program for Survivors of Torture — great hardships to go through that are difficult to talk about.

CHAPTER SIX

Balancing My Happiness against the Suffering of Others

My Health Worsens

I was hospitalized at Bellevue on May 23, 2003, for gangrene in my right ankle. Since then, neither antibiotics nor the daily curetting of the gangrene of my wound have helped the illness recede. The stench remains putrid. The analgesics, to ease the pain, are the only things that have a positive effect.

I consult more doctors, and they all draw the same fatal conclusion: amputation below the knee. My optimism is wearing down. In any case, I come to terms with my gullibility. No, the American care system is not almighty, despite all of its admirable achievements. The doctors cannot suggest any treatment that will bring my leg to life again. Rather, they invariably insist it is dead. They advise me against waiting any longer or else I risk needing to amputate not only below the knee but below the hip. According to them, the infection can only spread upward and become systemic. Eventually, I will die of septicemia, or blood poisoning.

As my health worsens, they seem to be right. During the month of August, I am overcome by abnormal fatigue. Though lying down all day, I am exhausted. Sleep no longer restores my energy. I wake up in the morning with a constantly intensifying feeling of weakness and breathlessness. X-rays reveal pleurisy, with pleura effusion, or inflammation and excess fluid in my chest cavity. That is not all. My whole body is giving out. I complain about acute and lingering lumbar pain, and I am diagnosed with Pott's disease, an infection of the vertebrae caused by tuberculosis. They put me on an IV of antibiotics.

My spine is so weakened that I have trouble straightening up. At times, I have to wear a stiff aluminum-and-polypropylene corset. It is a hard shell held by straps that keeps my spine straight. On the edge of the corset, there are rolls of foam supporting my arms under my armpits. The vertebrae are therefore decompressed because, thanks to the corset stretching out the spine, the weight supported by the lumbar vertebrae is relieved. I sometimes joke that I feel like the combination of several animals in one. With the corset, I look like a turtle with an artificial shell, and my gangrenous right foot resembles the leg of an elephant.

Today, I laugh when I think back on it. The turtle and the elephant became my totem animals as I lost my footing, both in a literal and a figurative sense. At the time, I could literally see my right foot decaying, and I lost my moral footing as well.

Every morning in the hospital, the curetting sessions continue, causing dreadful pain, and each time, the nurse extracts tiny pieces of bone. I now understand what the doctors mean when they talk about "destructive" arthritis. I am directly witnessing the disintegration of my body. My right foot looks more and more deathly, and the process is accelerating. There are increasing bone fragments in the purulent liquid that the nurses remove every day. The hope of seeing healthy tissue forming again is getting slimmer.

How is it possible not to imagine that a slow death by infection is spreading elsewhere in my skeleton? That my illness is about to generalize? I can see it in my foot. I cannot see it in my spine, but I am conscious that it is crumbling inexorably. On some days, I am not even able to sit down or stand up. I lose my balance with terrible pains, and I realize that, in such moments, my vertebrae are coming apart. I am doomed by the progress of my illness.

I am in psychological pain, too, for I am in a state of doubt. The pressure from the medical staff intensifies to make me accept amputation. They say that, once the problem of my foot is solved, they will be able to target the antibiotic therapy and concentrate on eradicating the tuberculosis of the bones. Yet each time I am tempted to accept amputation, an inner voice warns me insistently: *Don't amputate! Don't amputate!* But what if I have to cut my leg to live? I am disheartened by this inner conflict. I lose myself in conjectures.

In fact, I realize that I lost my footing, in a figurative sense, on the very day I landed on American soil. I believe this reveals a severe unsteadiness of the earth element in my inner mandala. Is it an effect of being uprooted? Some days I believe that I should take the plane back to India, if not to Tibet — that I should go back to a culture that I am familiar with, my monastery, my masters, and my family. My life as an exile is becoming unbearable for me. I am homesick for the country of my childhood and for the mountains that thrill me with their momentum toward the sky in a breathtaking cliff race.

Today, in a way that I wasn't aware of at the time, I believe that the turtle and the elephant were symbolic of an instinctive anchoring in the healing and protective energies of Mother Earth. These animals bear the world and humanity. They are emblems of wisdom, balance, stability, and longevity. While I was confronted with physical upheaval and inner chaos, they symbolized being rooted in the patience of the Earth. In retrospect, I may have unconsciously perceived a power of protection in these animals, and this may have helped me survive.

In the hospital, Marina tells me that America is called the "Island of the Turtle," since, according to Native American folklore, the weight of the continent rests on a turtle's back. In Tibet, the Gold Turtle spitting out fire is a sacred animal, an expression of awakened energy and of the foundation of the universe. Symbols of the astrological interpretation of the world are drawn on its belly. And the thrones of Buddha are carried by white elephants adorned with precious jewels.

Yet I am mostly haunted by the legend of the turtle and the floating sandalwood. In the Lotus Sutra, the Buddha explains how rare it is to encounter the Dharma with the analogy of how difficult it would be for a turtle to find a perfectly shaped piece of sandalwood floating on the surface of a big ocean. In the story, a turtle who has neither feet nor fins lives in the seabed. Its abdomen is as burning hot as if it were white-hot iron, and its shell is as cold as a mountain of ice. In such conditions, its only desire at all times, by day and by night, in the evening and in the morning, is to cool its belly and warm its shell.

It just so happens that red sandalwood has the power to cool its belly. This is sacred wood that, among all woods, resembles a wise man among men. The turtle, therefore, ardently wishes to haul itself up onto a floating piece of red sandalwood, one hollowed out exactly to fit its belly. Then it would be able to lay its belly on the wood to soothe the burning sensation, while the sun would warm its shell. But the laws of nature only allow this turtle to come to the surface of the water once every thousand years. And it is very difficult to find a floating piece of red sandalwood. The ocean is huge, the turtle very small, and floating pieces of sandalwood extremely rare. Supposing the turtle were lucky enough to discover one, there is a next to zero probability that the sandalwood would be hollowed in just the right way for the turtle. If the hollow were too big, the turtle would fall in and be stuck and shaded, and if the hollow were too small, the turtle would be carried away by the waves and fall back into the ocean. Such is the almost insurmountable challenge of encountering the Dharma, according to the Lotus Sutra.

In this difficult period of my life, am I not confronted with a similar dilemma? In the immeasurable ocean of world sufferings, with my gangrenous foot and my deteriorating vertebrae, I am the turtle without feet and fins. My body is subjected to dreadful pains, which sometimes give me the sensation of being branded, just like the turtle whose burning belly symbolizes the agonies of the eight hot hells. At other times, the pains make me shiver, just like the turtle suffering from its icy shell, which suggests the agonies endured in the eight cold hells.

The thousand years this reptile spends at the bottom of the ocean before resurfacing shows how difficult it is to be reborn as a human being. And right now, my mind is troubled by waves of despair and doubt, and I cannot enter deep meditation anymore. I often tell myself that, should I die in this situation, I would inevitably fall back down into the ocean just like the turtle, and it would take me a long time before being granted another precious human incarnation.

And yet, to extend the analogy, strapped up in the shell of my corset, I have found the sacred sandalwood of Dharma, which is so difficult to encounter on the surface of the vast ocean. But in my present situation, I am drifting. Assailed from all sides, there is great danger that the turmoil in my mind will overwhelm me. If I am not able to remain on my frail boat, I will end up like the turtle that, having miraculously found the sacred sandalwood, ends up unfortunately slipping and sinking to the seabed.

These thoughts add despair to despair. I do not sleep well, I have no appetite anymore, and I do not withstand pain as well. I cannot pray anymore. The days go by, and I sink into a sensation of unavoidable drowning. Even in jail I never had such a feeling of dejection. Pain and debasement remained external. I managed to stay upright. Torture did not wear down my capacity for resilience. Whereas at Bellevue Hospital, illness is killing me from the inside. As the days go by, I cannot hold back the psychological distress that accompanies my physical degeneration.

During the month of October, X-rays show, according to one report, a "completely destroyed ankle joint." The illness has become worse, and two months of antibiotic treatment have not gotten the better of the bone tuberculosis that is crushing the axis of my body. In this situation, what is the use of the daily curetting? It makes me suffer all the more because I do not see the point of it anymore. Then again, I am no longer in a position to refuse treatment. The medical staff has already given me an ultimatum. Either I accept the medical protocol and get ready for the operation, or I will have to end my hospitalization. I have been granted an extension to think about it, but I am afraid they will hasten my departure if I do not accept having my wound cleansed.

The nursing team has changed their attitude toward me. They are still kind when they speak to me, but I do not feel the same sympathy. I have been diagnosed as a tuberculosis germ carrier, so they protect themselves and come into my room wearing face masks. They also impose this measure on Marina. I can understand the reason for that. I don't want to contaminate anyone. However, how can I not feel plague-stricken, rejected, and excluded?

May I Be a Guard for Those Who Are Protectorless

For how long does this night of total sadness darken my mind? At least a week, and maybe two or even three. Withdrawn within my despair, I remain prostrate on my hospital bed, feeling homesick for my family and my monastery, which I think I will never see again.

The idea of dying in New York City is unbearable. I have already made inquiries. At Bellevue Hospital, the bodies of the deceased are laid in drawers in a refrigerated room before being buried in a communal grave for those who, like me, have neither family nor means. The mortuary seems to me the unavoidable antechamber of cold hells. Where will my mind go without being supported by prayers and rituals to guide it into the afterlife? I am terror-stricken.

On one of those desperate mornings, as a nurse is curetting my wound, removing the fragments of bone driven out by the purulent flesh, I suddenly recall this verse of the Indian saint Shantideva, which I learned very young at Golok Monastery:

May I be a guard for those who are protectorless,
A guide for those who journey on the road.
For those who wish to cross the water,
May I be a boat, a raft, a bridge.
May I be an isle for those who yearn for land,
A lamp for those who yearn for light,
For all who need a resting place, a bed.
For those who need a servant, may I be their slave.
May I be the wishing jewel, the vase of wealth,
A word of power, and the supreme healing,
May I be the tree of miracles,
For every being the abundant cow.
Just like the earth and space itself,
And all the other mighty elements,
For boundless multitudes of beings,
May I always be the ground of life, the source of varied
    sustenance.

I relax, and smile, despite the instrument digging into my open wound, despite the bad smell of blood and pus. From behind her mask, the nurse cries out. I do not understand what she is saying, but I can read her look. She is happy to see my face expressing peace after so many days of being unable to hide my despair.

I smile because I feel loved while mentally reciting these verses that express the pure state of the love of Buddhas. I feel loved, and I understand that, even hospitalized, disabled, in poor health, and contagious, even in this state, I can be loved, and I can love all beings, too. I realize that my body is admittedly seriously ill, but what about my mind?

My mind is not sick. Becoming aware of this is a giant step forward. For the first time in several weeks, I pray. I meditate on the radiant presence of awakened beings. I radiate their light toward all those who are suffering. From the bottom of my heart, I wish that Buddhas' blessings might support them as they cross the four rivers of suffering that torture beings, the rivers of birth, illness, old age, and death.

Lately, I have been obsessed by the fear of dying far from my loved ones. I have been thinking only of my own fate, my heart immured, my mind tortured by my inability to communicate. I at last manage to open up again! I feel liberated, and in a certain way, healed. I emerge from the prison I have let illness lock me into — an even worse dungeon than a prison cell, for it is inside myself! How could I have felt so sorry for myself to the point of inflicting on myself all these moral sufferings?

I think of others who are less fortunate, who do not have access to medical treatment. I have seen the living conditions among the homeless people north of Delhi, in the Indian quarter adjoining the Tibetan colony of Majnu Ka Tilla, on the banks of the Yamuna River. Every day, some die in utter destitution, of illness, of malnutrition, of heat during the dry season, or of cold during winter. In the early morning, the police are on the beat. Specialized teams wrap corpses into plastic bags before throwing them into a dump truck, with no respect, no humanity. While I am enjoying regular treatment and constant care in this American hospital. How can I have been so selfish? How can I have wasted all these days thinking only of myself, feeling sorry for myself, when so many would envy my lot?

I pray fervently:

May beings everywhere who suffer
Torment in their minds and bodies
Have, by virtue of my merit,
Joy and happiness in boundless measure.

Balancing My Own Happiness Against the Suffering of Others

Marina has been asking me for a long time to do some teaching. She has introduced me to other PhD students under Robert Thurman who are fascinated by Buddhist philosophy and spirituality. I choose to transmit a short text, *The Thirty-Seven Verses on the Practice of a Bodhisattva*, which is the essence of sublime instructions on the Heart of Compassion.

So it is that, the first time I teach in the West, it is from a hospital bed. I speak to people wearing masks to avoid the risk of contamination. But their eyes are nonetheless watchful and filled with emotion, as I try to sow the leaven of great loving compassion into their stream of consciousness.

Bodhisattvas are beings who have awakened from ignorance. With the gift of their benevolent love, they create the causes of happiness for all beings, and through their compassion, they deliver them from suffering. Love and compassion: These words take on a new shape after the painful experience of the previous weeks. I now feel intimately linked with the beings who experience suffering in all realms of existence. I can perceive the awakening dimension of love and compassion. These strengths allow change and are capable of transforming ordinary people into bodhisatt-vas. I was revealed their secret as I experienced the kind of pain that sanctifies you. As it is said in this verse from *The Thirty-Seven Verses on the Practice of a Bodhisattva*:

All suffering without exception arises from desiring
    happiness for oneself,
While perfect buddhahood is born from the thought of
    benefiting others.
Therefore, to really exchange my own happiness for the
    sufferings of others
Is the practice of a Bodhisattva.

Reading these words, compassion is like a river of joy run-ning through me. Overflowing from my heart, it absorbs the painful feelings of my body, and I can feel its healing energy. It uproots the self-centered experience of the world, where percep-tion of reality, distorted by uncontrolled instincts, is the cause of deep suffering. I have always heard my masters describe the ego as an "evil monster" and say:

All the violence, all the perils, all the sufferings of the
    world
Come from attachment to our ego.
What have you got to do with this harmful monster?
If you don't give up your self, you will continue endlessly
    to suffer,
In the same way as when you don't draw your hand away
    from fire,
You cannot avoid it being burned.

A bodhisattva's love welcomes the sufferings of beings in an unconditional way. That is when the boundless field of nondual-istic experience opens up, once the mind is awakened to its true nature. Then, compassion meets wisdom, for on an ultimate level, love perfectly realizes the deep interdependent links that unite all lives.

So it is that, twenty years later and seventy-five hundred miles away, I recall the fervor of the dream that drew me to the pure lands of the Maitreya Buddha and Je Tsongkhapa. After over four months of intense physical and moral suffering, I renew the offering of my life to all beings:

> May beings everywhere who suffer
> Torment in their minds and bodies
> Have, by virtue of my merit,
> Joy and happiness in boundless measure....
> May beings never suffer anguish
> Let them not be sick or evilly behave.
> May they have no fear, nor suffer insults,
> Always may their minds be free from sorrow....
> May the blind receive their sight,
> And may the deaf begin to hear,
> And women near their time bring forth,
> Like Mayadevi, free from all travail....
> May the naked now be clothed,
> And all the hungry eat their fill,
> And may those parched with thirst receive
> Pure waters and delicious drinks....
> May the poor and destitute find wealth,
> The haggard and the careworn, joy.
> May those now in despair be whole in mind,
> Endowed with sterling constancy....
> May kindly spirits bring the rains on time,
> For harvests to be rich and plentiful....
> May medicines be full of strength,
> May secret words of power be chanted with success....

May every being ailing with disease
Be freed at once from every malady.
May every sickness that afflicts the living
Be wholly and forever absent from the world....
May those who go in dread have no more fear.
May captives be unchained and now set free.
And may the weak receive their strength.
May living beings help each other in kindness....

PART THREE

MEDITATION AND HEALING

Appearances and emptiness inseparable are like the empty sky;
People of Tingri, the mind is without either center or periphery.

— PADAMPA SANGYE

CHAPTER SEVEN

Why Do You Seek Healing outside of Yourself?

My Letter to the Dalai Lama

It is November 2003, and the doctors' ultimatum is about to expire. During this fall in New York City, after six months of treatment at Bellevue Hospital, my condition has only worsened. The gangrene, as purulent as ever, is still crumbling the bones of my right ankle. The latest X-ray reports show that the talus is now completely destroyed. The disease is starting to erode the base of the tibia. The antibiotic therapy, unable to limit its progression, has checked neither the pleurisy nor the bone tuberculosis. In such conditions, it would be more reasonable to follow the doctors' recommendations and accept amputation. However, the inner voice continues to warn me. I have to refuse this operation.

Physical mutilation is disabling. But another problem comes with it. Cutting part of my leg also means destroying the physical support of the corresponding subtle nervous system. Later on, this will be an obstacle in my practices of inner energy yoga because, at advanced stages, they require being able to make the vital principle circulate throughout a complete physical body. During the process of death, it is also necessary for the network of channels and chakras to be as intact as possible. Our consciousness leaves our body through one of its nine doors — which include the door to Brahma on the fontanel and the upper and lower orifices. But only the crown chakra at the top of the head is a "white" door; the others are "black" doors, since they open onto rebirth in lower realms of existence. To manage to eject one's consciousness from the top, the vital principle energy must not be off course or blocked. Hence the importance of preserving the integrity of the subtle body, and therefore that of the correlated physical body.

Filled with questions like that, I receive very favorably a suggestion by Marina. She tells me that Robert Thurman is leaving for Dharamsala in two days. Marina has told Bob about me, and if it is my wish, he has agreed to deliver a message from me to the Dalai Lama. I could explain my situation to him and beseech him to give me advice on what decision to make.

The Dalai Lama is my source of refuge in this life, and in all of my lives. When I wake up in the morning, I visualize him above my head, diffusing an aura of kindness that brightens up my day. In the evening, I beseech him to come down onto the cup of the lotus on my heart chakra. I close up the petals around this sacred light, which illuminates me from the inside. The prayer for the Dalai Lama, who is the incarnation of the Buddha of Compassion in our world, is with me day and night. His presence within me has already helped me go through the most painful moments of my life in prison, and it supports me in the ordeal I am going through now at Bellevue Hospital. I am serene and relieved to be able to leave this decision to him.

Though I feel an urgency to write to Kundun, the letter has to conform to a strict etiquette. For this very particular letter, I appeal to Pema Dorje. Through Thinley, this monk has already heard about me within the Tibetan community in New York City, and I am always delighted when he comes to visit me. He makes me delicious vegetarian *momos*, a type of Tibetan steamed ravioli, and brings me roasted barley flour with yak cheese. Not only do I appreciate these dishes, which are a change from the ordinary bland fare at the hospital, but his jolly and warm company is a great comfort. At this point, he is the first and only monk that I have met in New York City. His story is symbolic of the Tibetan diaspora, which has been marked for two generations by loss, separation, and the mourning of loved ones through all sorts of cruel events.

About ten years older than me, Pema Dorje was born in a nomadic family on the Roof of the World on the high steppes of Ngari, in western Tibet along the Ladakh border. His parents owned big droves of yaks and horses and flocks of sheep; every year, his father, Ngangurk, would lead a little caravan to Nepal. He used to swap salt harvested on the banks of brackish lakes, butter, and tightly knit yak wool materials for rice, corn, millet, chili, and paper. Pema has wonderful memories of his birthplace, an imposing area where rocks pray, icily guarded by Khang Rinpoche, the "precious jewel of snow," a Tibetan nickname for Mount Kailash. He recalls Lake Manasarovar, a fascinating mirror of the fleeting clouds sailing through the cobalt blue sky. It was nicknamed Mapham Tso, "The Invincible," for this lake is said to collect in its holy waters the omnipotence of the omniscient mind, which conquers illusory phenomena.

Threatened by the People's Liberation Army, Pema's family had to leave these celestial expanses in 1960, entrusting their animals to the care of an elderly aunt and her son. But they were intercepted by Chinese patrols on their way to exile. Pema's father and his two uncles were imprisoned. Only his father survived the horrors of detention. Liberated a year later, he joined his family, who were gathered with other nomads in loathsome jails. Living conditions were dreadful, and food and hygiene were appalling. His parents died within a week of each other. On her deathbed,

Pema's mother made him promise to treat all beings with equal kindness and compassion. She made the wish that her son might attempt at all cost to reach Dharamsala, in India, to receive a Buddhist education with the Dalai Lama and become a monk. In 1975, at the age of twenty-two, Pema applied to enter Nechung Monastery, the headquarters of the State Oracle of Tibet exiled in Dharamsala. Later, in 1994, he took refuge in New York City. By the time I met him, he had become the secretary of the Nechung Foundation and the principal of the Sunday school dedicated to the New York and New Jersey Tibetan community.

Pema Dorje and I feel very close right away. More than both being monks, we are deeply united by the resilience we have forged through hardships. Unlike other Tibetans, who are haunted by hatred and anger, we feel tremendous compassion for our Chinese brothers and sisters. But there is also more to it. Our links go further back than our present lives.

Throughout my reincarnations, the destinies of the Phakyab Rinpoches and of the Nechung Oracles have come across one another in unusual circumstances. The abbey of Nechung Monastery is also the Dalai Lama's private oracle, and he holds the rank of vice-minister in the exiled Tibetan government. As the holder of secret tantric transmissions, he is considered a *ku-ten*, the physical embodiment in human shape of a spirit who receives messages and predictions when in a trance. "I ask for advice from the oracle as I would consult my staff or my conscience," the Dalai Lama once admitted.

My previous incarnation, the seventh Phakyab Rinpoche, happened to be in Lhasa in the winter of 1926. Then thirty-three years old, he had made a pilgrimage to the holy city. As the Thirteenth Dalai Lama was teaching initiations at Drepung Monastery, Phakyab Rinpoche sat down anonymously among a crowd of more than seven thousand monks. Wearing the garments of a wandering yogi, he looked no different than the others, but the Nechung Oracle recognized him at first sight. He bowed in front of him and paid him tribute, calling him Rigpa Zinpa, "holder of the clear light of the heart." Inviting Rinpoche to follow him, the Oracle escorted him to the platform, where he was offered a high seat at the foot of the "Ocean of Wisdom."

Eight decades later, in this early winter of 2003, I am far from Tibet. In a New York hospital, a monk from Nechung comes to my bedside. This time, it is to write a message to be delivered to the Fourteenth Ocean of Wisdom. Karma makes light of times and locations, weaving the invisible threads of what we call fate.

I am happy to see Pema Dorje appear in the doorway. Not very tall, but broad-shouldered, his triangular face with high cheekbones is lit up by the benevolent love he has for all beings with equanimity. He has remained a monk in the United States, but he only wears his monk's dress for religious rites and community celebrations. By day, he works hard on building sites and prefers wearing civilian clothes. I make a different choice. I am still wearing my monastic clothes, despite the pressure from Thinley to leave them in a cupboard as soon as I had arrived. It is true that walking with crutches was not easy, and my dress was no help. I had to be very careful to not stumble. Also, people noticed me a lot more in this getup, and Thinley was embarrassed by all the people turning around as we went by.

But my monk's dress means a lot more to me than simple clothes. I received it with my ordination, and it symbolizes offering my life for all beings. In this outfit, I am clothed with the blessings of the Buddhas, whose spirit of love radiates on others. At the hospital, I put on my crimson dress over my saffron shirt every morning, despite the recommendations of nurses who praise the better comfort of hospital gowns.

If Pema Dorje does not look like a monk, he embodies a

monk's qualities of peace, perfect humility, and joy. I called him last night, and he has come to see me this afternoon, since it is Monday and his day off. Together we prepare the wording of my letter to the Dalai Lama. We address him with the set formulas expressing our devotion: "Holy Compassionate Lord," "Gentle Glory," "Wish-Fulfilling Jewel," and "Precious Conqueror." To begin, Pema Dorje copies down a devout prayer, paying tribute to all the uncommon realizations of Kundun in the flourishing style of Buddhist sutras:

> Om Svasti! You embody the wisdom, the love, and the strength of all Buddhas and omniscient Bodhisattvas, showing all their attributes and signs in your perfect and complete shape.
>
> You are compassion itself, Holder of the Padmapani Lotus, in the shape of a saffron-dressed monk. Supreme guide, ambassador of peace in the world, sole protector of the Tibetan people, omniscient Lord of victories, Tenzin Gyatso, I pay tribute to your body, your speech, and your mind filled with devotion!
>
> Because you reveal yourself in this "World of Suffering" in the shape of a perfect Buddha, bringing into play the wisdom of renunciation and realization, the ocean of scholars and siddhas supporting the traditions of sutras and tantras is gathered before you, eager to serve you promptly.
>
> All the people in high places of the three realms of this world, filled with fervor, want to contemplate your noble face, to hear your eloquent words. On all continents, your influence shines in all directions, victorious among all, you are unequalled.

We then state my question in simple and direct words. First, we recall that, in 1994, Kundun officially recognized me as the eighth Phakyab Rinpoche, holder of the Ashi throne. Last April 26, I took off for the United States with his blessing. At my arrival, I was diagnosed with incurable gangrene on the right foot. Should I accept amputation of the leg below the knee, or should I seek another treatment?

Once drafted, and reread several times, Pema Dorje — who excels at calligraphy — writes the message in gold ink on beautiful light green organic paper, which he has brought for this occasion. I append my signature, and the envelope is ready when Marina comes to pick it up later that afternoon. She is going to give it personally to Robert Thurman, who is flying off to Dharamsala the next morning.

The answer is not long coming. Five days later, on November 16, Marina gets a phone call from Robert Thurman, and then she calls me. My heart is pounding as she delivers the Dalai Lama's message. Since a terrible thunderstorm is raging at the same time over Manhattan, I have to ask her to repeat the message several times. Each word is engraved in my memory for life.

"Why do you seek healing outside of yourself?" asks Kundun. "You have within you the wisdom that heals, and once healed, you will teach the world how to heal."

In Tibetan, the message is twenty-five words long.

Twenty-five words seal my fate.

There are other instructions recommending beneficial practices, as well as the appropriate visualizations and mantras to chant.

Illnesses Caused by Spirits

Kundun does not tell me to refuse amputation. He tests me. He questions me. I have been turning this question over and over again in my mind for weeks. I came to the United States convinced that the sophisticated American health system should easily cure a man like me, in the prime of life, hardened by a rough but healthy lifestyle on the high plateaus. How is it possible that Western civilization, which masters so many fabulous techniques, would not know how to treat the problem with my ankle? It has taken me a few months to understand that such is not the case.

"Why do you seek healing outside of yourself?"

When my inner voice first told me not to accept amputation, I obviously listened to it, since I refused the protocol for the operation that the doctors were urging me to accept. But I did not go deeper into the subject. I did not try to understand where this voice was coming from, nor what it was revealing to me. I did this precisely because I was expecting to be healed from the outside, a providential healing. I was expecting everything from Western science.

Now I am admitting that the pathology I am suffering from is beyond existing treatments. From a medical point of view, my illness is incurable. Moreover, my caretakers have given up hope for me. From the beginning, they have not ceased repeating that my ankle is dead; that if I wait any longer, my leg will die; and that, if this happens, I will end up dying. Such is the external and physiological dimension of my illness. It is supported and confirmed by X-rays, tissue analysis, and blood tests. This picture is final. It is a death warrant.

"Why do you seek healing outside of yourself?"

In asking me this question, the Dalai Lama reminds me that, if my gangrene cannot be taken care of by the hospital, it does not imply that it is incurable. It is not fatal. It can be treated, or even healed, by using a treatment protocol that is not only physical. Kundun is urging me to become aware of the true nature of my illness.

Pema Dorje has told me about the tragic case of a young monk from Namgyal, the Dalai Lama's private monastery. His first name was also Pema, and he was the Dalai Lama's favorite artist. He was brilliant; he spoke and wrote English perfectly. He had studied under Robert Thurman and had been awarded a master's degree at Columbia University in New York City. Then he was suddenly affected by a serious health problem, a tumor in the lung. In addition to consulting Western doctors, Pema consulted Tibetan doctors, who recommended not to operate. They diagnosed that the cause of the illness was not physical. It was provoked by nagas, the spirits of water. Pema had taken part in the ritual consecrating the temple dedicated to them in the Dalai Lama's residence in Dharamsala. Perhaps he had unconsciously offended these very irritable beings, who suffer intensely nowadays because of environmental pollution and deforestation, as watercourses and trees are their abodes.

Pema was undoubtedly too confident in the American health system, as I had been when I arrived at Bellevue Hospital. The doctors suspected cancer and urged him to accept an operation. Once the tumor was removed, a biopsy showed that it was benign, but the damage had been done. To remove these fibrous tissues, the doctors had to cut out a piece of trachea. Pema underwent a total of five invasive surgeries, and a piece of intestine was used to reconstruct the trachea. He died of complications following these operations.

Before Pema died, Robert Thurman went to visit him in the intensive care unit. On the eve of his death, with an exemplary strength of soul, he was still joyful and joking. He asked Bob to save his scholarship for him. He said he would need it in his next reincarnation, when he would come back to Columbia University to resume writing his dissertation for his PhD!

"Why do you seek healing outside of yourself?"

Just like Pema, the cause of my illness might be internal. When the Tibetan doctors advised him against operating, they

urged Pema to do a spiritual retreat, with specific mantra chanting. When people are affected by the nagas, it corresponds to
an unbalance of the water element on an energetic level, and of
phlegm mucus on a physical level. Thanks to propitiatory rituals,
natural harmony is reestablished and allows for healing.

In Tibet, I practiced a lot of rituals to the nagas, for the spirits
of rivers, and nature in general, are suffering terribly from the environmental exploitation of the Chinese. Later, Robert Thurman
will ask me to come every year to Menla Mountain, a Dharma
sanctuary in the Catskills, New York, for a ritual to the great naga
inhabiting the premises. The Dalai Lama blessed it during one of
his visits. I will glimpse it, too. One day, it will poke its enormous
head through my window frame, then leave as swiftly as a breath
of air.

Nanda Entering the Womb Sutra

The story of Pema, the Namgyal monk, makes me reflect. I recall the teaching given by the Buddha to Prince Nanda, his half-
brother. The young man was bewitched by the beauty of his wife,
Janapada Kalyani. He only had eyes for her, whose sensual grace
outshone all courtesans, and she filled him with bliss. In order
to distract his attention from the pleasures of samsara — which
cause innumerable afflictions — and to guide him onto the spiritual path, the Awakened explained to him all the endless sufferings of conditioned existence. This is the subject of the sermon
called "Nanda Entering the Womb Sutra."

According to this teaching, torments start at the very moment of conception, when the consciousness of the baby to be
born merges with the father-mother cells. It then feels as if it were
diving into a huge cauldron, boiling with the heat of hot hells.
In the following weeks, the formation of the head and the four
limbs causes a sensation of stretching that is as painful as being

quartered on the torture wheel. Within the womb, as it develops, the fetus is oppressed, suffocating, crushed as if under enormous rocks. Its disgust for the foul mugginess of its abode does not cease to get worse as the weeks go by, for space becomes more and more limited. At birth, it feels caught in the vaginal stranglehold. In the sutra, the Buddha goes on to describe the drawbacks of conditioned existence by introducing the four categories of illnesses that will affect the newborn as soon as he or she comes into the world.

The first ones, benign, will spontaneously heal. For the second ones, more severe, there are treatments, and the patient recovers. A third category of ailments has no therapeutic response. All remedies are doomed to fail, but it is still possible to cure with spiritual practices. Finally, the last category of illness is irreversible. Linked with the karma of death, the outcome is fatal despite remedies and treatments. Taking medicine, to no avail, might even increase the pain by disrupting the natural process with which the consciousness leaves the body.

"Why do you seek healing outside of yourself?"

This question makes me reflect. What type of illness am I suffering from? At this point, no medical protocol has been effective. I have tried everything. In India, at this point, I might have thought there still would be a stroke of salvation left if I could access Western medicine. But these last six months in New York City have proven that is not the case. The karmic causes of my illness are such that they do not respond to existing medical treatments. If I am to believe Kundun's message, there is still some hope that the causes are not drastic enough to lead me to death. My illness belongs therefore to the third category. I have reasons to believe that its origin is blended with the mysteries of my reincarnations. I must seek for them in the spiritual memory of my lineage.

At the Age of Twenty-Eight,
I Am Twelve Hundred Years Old

During the spring of 1994, I am involved in long studies, a curriculum in philosophy alternating with meditative retreats. It takes about twenty years to achieve the respected degree of Geshe Lharampa. Translated into U.S. academic terms, this is approximately equivalent to a PhD in divinity, even if the American degree does not include the meditative dimension. But the level of studies in philosophy and psychology is considered to be equivalent.

At Sera Mey Monastery, in the state of Karnataka near Mysore, I spend my days studying and praying. My masters are gentle, considerate, and great yogis filled with kindness. Some of them are awakened monks that nobody notices, so humble and discreet they are. Their level of realization is often discovered only after their death. This was the case with one of my masters, Geshe Lodro. He remained during fifteen days in *tukdam*, or death meditation. It was the hot season, reaching a stifling 104° F or more in our tiny living quarters, with neither fan nor air-conditioning. However, despite such heat, his physical body did not decay. Rays of light and fragrances came from it. Only when he broke his *tukdam* did his tissues start to putrefy very quickly. After his cremation, relics were found among his ashes, a great number of *rinsel* — little white iridescent pearls that are the ultimate blessings of awakened beings at the end of their life on Earth.

Since 1985, I have been studying with these immensely kind masters, though living conditions are difficult for lack of food. There is often only a cup of tea with milk for breakfast, a little bowl of rice with lentils for lunch, and our supper is limited to half a piece of bread. We are all skinny, and our ears, on both sides of our wasted faces, seem disproportionately big. Once, when one of my roommates falls ill, I take care of him at the request of my master, but my own fate worsens, for I do not have enough time to appear at the refectory on time. After evening prayers, since I'm forced to skip the meager meals of the monastery, I vainly try to warm and soften potatoes in the palms of my hands. I end up eating them raw, since I'm not able to cook them. In times like these, I sometimes shed tears of nostalgia thinking of the meals my mother would prepare with such love. Yet, despite the hunger churning in my stomach, my mind is joyful and in peace. I do not feel the need for entertainment, and I devote most of my time to studying or meditating following the benevolent instructions of my masters.

Now, I am about to turn twenty-eight, and I am preparing to take the end-of-year exams before the rainy season starts in June. That is when the abbey sends for me to come to his apartment, adjacent to the assembly room. I prostrate myself three times before him, as is the custom. He sits on the high bed that he uses as a throne by day and as a bed by night. On the other side of the partition wall, the monks are chanting the evening prayers. I raise my eyes questioningly, curious to know the reason why he has summoned me. His hatchet face brightens up with a big smile.

He puts on his glasses and reads to me, articulating each word, a letter on which I recognize the red ink seal of the Dalai Lama. Kundun declares that, on request of the monks at Ashi in Lithang, he has looked for the new incarnation of the seventh Phakyab Rinpoche, holder of the throne of their monastery. The necessary prayers and divinations have revealed that the eighth reincarnation, bearing the name of Yeshi Dorje, is a boy born in the valley of Nyagchu, on the tenth day of the fifth month in the year of the Fire Goat — meaning June 24, 1966, in the Western calendar. His mother's name is Sonam Dolma. Yeshi Dorje was ordained monk under the name of Lobsang Dhondup and is currently studying at Sera Mey.

When I hear the exact day of my birth, my name, my mother's

name, the name of my valley, and my name as a monk, I under-
stand that the letter is about me. However, it is as if the abbey were
talking about another when he announces: "Your title is Phakyab
Rinpoche. The name of the reincarnated spiritual master that
His Holiness the Dalai Lama has given you is Ngawang Sungrab
Tenzin Gelek Gyatso, 'Powerful Voice — Awakened Speech —
Holder of the Dharma and of Virtue — Victorious Ocean.'"

I remain silent, dumbfounded, stupefied, gazing into emptiness. The abbey asks me if I have a question. Before I say a word,
he expresses his joy at saluting the eighth Phakyab Rinpoche and
offers me his best wishes in the fulfillment of my mission: "The
Phakyab Rinpoches are famous masters. You hold the lineage of
transference of consciousness at the time of death, and of appease-
ment of suffering through the noble perfection of wisdom. You
are currently one of the best students at Sera Mey, a humble and
very pure monk. It is excellent for you to continue your studies
until you reach the Geshe Lharampa degree, and with Kundun's
blessings, you will awaken a great number of beings. I pay tribute
to the eighth Phakyab Rinpoche, a lion among men."

I answer dully that I am happy with my lot. Having all I could
wish for in my life as a monk, and in my studies at the monastery,
I wish for nothing more. The abbey laughs and states that he will
give me some time to think it over. We will talk about it again in a
few days, after my exams.

As I go back to my room, warm drops of rain start falling
down, soft and round. This shower, ahead of the monsoon,
brings a freshness to soothe the burning sensation of the day. It
also calms down the great turmoil that the news of my recogni-
tion by His Holiness has caused in my mind. I let the water soak
my cheeks. The rain, in these moments, seems like a sign from
the sky and a blessing from the dakinis. These deities, mothers of
space, patrons of yogis, are inviting me to rejoice over the happy

accomplishment of karma. But the joy and the celebration of my investiture will come later. For the time being, I choose to go back to my studies and concentrate on revising. I am deeply satisfied with the fifteen years spent in monasteries in Tibet and in South India. I do not, in the slightest way, want to bear the responsibilities of a rinpoche.

That is what I state, with some boldness, three weeks later, when the abbey summons me again. I have brilliantly succeeded in my exams, and I declare that I want to continue in this way. Having reached the degree of Geshe, I will be able to teach unsparingly the Dharma and work to liberate beings from suffering. This time the superior puts on a stern look. He hands me Kundun's letter and drily declares: "You answer the Dalai Lama yourself, telling him you have been informed, and that, with full knowledge of the facts, you renounce being the eighth Phakyab Rinpoche."

The abbey of Sera Mey has put me in front of my fate. I dared say no to him. But I obviously cannot say no to Kundun.

My life suddenly takes on several lives.

At the age of twenty-eight, I am twelve hundred years old.

Padampa Sangye, the First in My Lineage of Reincarnation

The history of incarnated time is a whispered memory, transmitted from mind to mind. Many a unique and priceless manuscript was destroyed during the Cultural Revolution. Or they have not made it to the land of exile, India. As such, we do not have, in written form, all the biographies of the previous Phakyab Rinpoches. These texts, written in the flourished, ornamented style of hagiography, are called *namtar* in Tibetan, or "liberating life story."* Not being able to find a *namtar* of the previous holders

---

* The literal translation of *namtar* from Tibetan is "complete liberation."

of my lineage, I thus went to see an old monk at Sera Mey who had been, as a child, the servant of the seventh Phakyab Rinpoche at Ashi Monastery. He gave me information on the story of my reincarnations. He felt tremendous devotion for my predecessor. Shedding tears that got lost in the furrows of his wrinkles, he told me how the seventh Phakyab Rinpoche had to disappear and hide to escape the terrible persecutions that struck eastern Tibet in the 1950s. He died as a yogi recluse in the secrecy of a solitary cave, and that is when the monk who'd been his servant decided to join the Dalai Lama in exile in India.

As far as the memory of my lineage goes back, I was born for the first time in the year 740 in central India. I was one of the pundits of the Nalanda monastery, ordained under the name of Kamalashila when, at the request of King Trisong Detsen, I went to Tibet. At Samye Monastery,* I defeated — in a verbal joust that remains famous in history — the Chinese master Heshang Moheyan, leader of the Northern Chan School, who was spreading false views on the Dharma. While I was officiating as master of the rituals, Padmasambhava asked me to go teach the doctrine of Buddha in China. I then spent eighty years in the Middle Kingdom to purify the erroneous interpretations of the Dharma that ignorant masters were preaching.

When I deemed my task accomplished, I made it known that I wanted to leave. But my disciples did not want to hear about it. They bribed the ferryman so that he would not take me to the other bank of the river. As I was trying to escape in a hasty departure, I lost one of my sandals, and when I reached the ford, the ferryman declared there was no ferryboat. I then placed a water lily leaf on the water, set my feet on it, and used it as a frail boat.

---

* Samye Monastery is one of the oldest monasteries in Tibet, consecrated by Padmasambhava in 779.

The goddess mounted on a tiger issued from the wisdom eye on her forehead a magical red-coated mare that took my sandal between her teeth and brought it back to me in a flash.

I was thus, in this first incarnation, a Mahasiddha, or "Great Accomplished," initiated into all the mandalas of the tantric tradition of Diamond Way Buddhism. Endowed with the armor of compassion, and cherishing others more than myself, I was deeply beneficial to those who approached me throughout my life. If we are to believe certain mystical tales, I must have revealed the *siddhi* of immortality and lived 572 years.

It is when I appeared again in Tibet after the year 1113, and after my journey to China, that Tibetans gave me the name of Padampa Sangye. My physical appearance had by then completely changed. This involuntary transformation occurred as I was going through a valley where the body of an elephant was blocking a river. His body had started to decay, which risked infecting the river, thereby causing an epidemic among the villagers. A sadhu, an Indian ascetic or renouncer, named Dampa Nagchung, or the "Black Dampa," lived nearby. He asked me if I would transfer my consciousness into this elephant, then climb toward a rocky, desert area nearby where vultures would come devour the elephant. Dampa Nagchung promised to keep an eye on my body while I inhabited the body of the elephant, and upon returning, I would find my body intact. I accepted and obliged him, happy to be able to spare the farmers and their herd all risk of infection.

While I was climbing toward the heights in the body of the elephant, Dampa Nagchung could not resist the temptation to exchange his ugly old body for my sound and healthy one. Since he was a yogi and accomplished in the art of transferring consciousness, he did so, and when I came back, I found only the corpse of the sadhu on the riverbank. I was repulsed by his remains, and I hesitated to reincarnate into his shape. I thought it better to go to the pure lands. But a dakini sang in my ear a song of ecstasy, which persuaded me to take on the body of Dampa Nagchung, since my mission on Earth was not finished.

I then reincarnated, and the celestial dakini guided me toward the banks of the Arun, one of the rare Tibetan rivers whose waters pierce a hole into the Himalayan barrier before streaming down to the plains of Nepal. Going through this area where the air is as pure as crystal, I stopped at Tingri and stayed there for twenty years. The people of Tingri gave me the name "Black Padampa Buddha," since I had the dark skin of the Indian sadhu who had stolen my body.

At Tingri, the dakini had announced to me that I would accomplish a miraculous karma. For the Shakyamuni Buddha, at the time when he was teaching the Sutra of the Perfection of Wisdom at Vulture Peak, had thrown a stone very high in the air toward the north. He had prophesied that, at the very spot where it would fall down, a master in the future would come transmit these same sutras, which contain the essence of Awakening. The stone had reached the top of a hill, the only bulging spot on the smooth and arid surface of the plateau where I was, blocked off in the distance by the snowy peaks of Mount Everest. Upon hitting the hill, a "ting" sound had strongly resonated all around, and that is why the inhabitants named this hamlet Tingri.

Following the dakini's instructions, I found the blessed stone near a stupa. As I touched it, as if by magic, a musk deer — which had ritually turned around the stupa several times — was absorbed in it. I therefore taught, for several months, the Sutra of the Perfection of Wisdom, and once the prophecy was achieved, I left my body.

A few decades later, I appeared again in the form of Tiphupa, who was the reincarnation of Darma Dodde, son and disciple of

Marpa, Milarepa's master, who awakened in the twelfth century. At the age of sixteen, I had a riding accident and I was brought back to my father in a state of unconsciousness. He managed to keep me alive for a few hours, the time needed to teach me the practice of transference of consciousness, or *powa* in Tibetan, a practice also called "opening the door to the sky." I looked around for a deceased human body to transfer my consciousness into, but found none. There was only, nearby, the body of a pigeon. I blended my mind with the remains of this animal and took off toward the blessed land of India.

I flew over the Himalayas and, near Varanasi, the luminous city on the banks of the Ganges, I saw weeping parents watching over their sixteen-year-old son, a Brahman who had just died. I transferred my consciousness into him and became a famous master of *powa*, which is when I was given the Tibetan name of Tiphupa, "Lord Pigeon." Later, I went back to Tibet to take care of my parents in their old age. I carried on the teaching tradition of my father, Marpa. One of my students was Rechungpa, a close disciple of Milarepa.

In Bellevue Hospital, as I recall in detail the uncommon accomplishments of the first holders of my lineage, it is hard to admit that the mind of these awakened beings lives in the ordinary and gangrenous monk I have become today! In such moments, like when the secret of my reincarnation was revealed to me, I tell myself that only the blessings of the Dalai Lama, and an intense practice of compassion for the wellness of all beings, will help me transcend my limits and heal, if I do have this healing karma. As for my illness, it is obvious to me that it is not separate from the story of my lineage.

I often recall that my predecessor, the seventh Phakyab Rinpoche, had a weakness in his right leg. At the end of his life, he was the "lama with an elephant foot," as I am today, bedridden in a New York City hospital. When he decided to leave his body at the age of sixty-two, he let this health issue deteriorate, though he had managed to control it until then, and he died within a few days of what today is called deep vein thrombosis.

Am I going to die if I do not accept amputation?

Probably not, if I go by the Dalai Lama's message. However, I am not unaware of the fact that the doctors have formally warned me. I see fear in their eyes. As for myself, I am not worried. I have already risked dying quite often in this life, such as when I was imprisoned, and then when I crossed the Himalayan passes three times. And in the unfathomable abysses of time, I have been born and died an incalculable number of times. In my everyday practices, I die and am born again six times a day. In meditation, I have experimented with the process through which consciousness separates from its physical support and remerges with it.

More than ever, at Bellevue Hospital, I feel that death expresses the impermanence of phenomena. It is inscribed in time, the internal dimension of the world, animate as well as inanimate. There is no life without death. Meditating on death means meditating on life. In this great cycle of transformation, death is one of the four phases of the process, which starts with the beginning of life and birth, followed by growth and maturity, then decline, and at last destruction or death — before a new rebirth.

Being born and dying come together. The beginning and the end of life, apparently opposite, form a continuity of events of consciousness. Such is the movement of the Wheel of Time, affecting all that appears in the universe, from the sand grain to the galaxies, from the infinitesimal to the infinitely great. As the eighth in my lineage, I can feel the deep psychological union that goes beyond the boundaries of my physical life — similar to an immaterial river, flowing from mind to mind from time immemorial. The impression of dying is only the result of an incomplete vision, and I meditate the essence of the mind beyond birth and death.

What If My Illness Were a Blessing?

"You have within you the wisdom that heals."

These words of the Dalai Lama urge me to meditate an uncommon wisdom: the wisdom of the inconceivable, the wisdom embracing the universe. I have been initiated by my masters, and I have been prepared for it by the real-life experience of my childhood. Reaching that level of consciousness implies entering a boundless dimension at the very root of Buddha's teaching.

In the sixteenth chapter of the Lotus Sutra, Buddha upsets his audience. His contemporaries all believe he has achieved illumination at Bodhgaya.

"You are quite mistaken, says the Blessed. I have been awakened since a time without beginning. Trying to grasp this extremely remote length of time in your temporal unit of time measurement is vain. There is neither birth nor death, neither withdrawal nor emergence, no one to reside in the world nor to end up disappearing."

When Buddha leaves his body in Kushinagar, it is an ultimate attempt to urge his disciples to undertake their own quest for the path. To make them understand that, if he remained in this world of illusion, few of them would realize how necessary it is to put his teachings into practice, Buddha resorts to the Parable of the Excellent Physician. A renowned doctor is away, and during his trip abroad, his sons inadvertently swallow poisoned food. Upon returning, the father immediately prepares the antidote that will save them. While some of his sons take it, and are immediately cured, others, despite dreadful pain, stubbornly refuse to take the remedy. The doctor thus uses a clever means. He sends a messenger bearing the news of his death. In the grip of sorrow and fear, the rebellious sons drink the potion and are saved. In the same way, without ever moving away from us, the Buddha uses the emptiness caused by his absence to divert those who go astray on wrong paths. He then emerges to teach the Dharma, once their frame of mind has adjusted.

The true nature of Buddha is altogether universal and timeless. That is why the Blessed claims to have reached Awakening for a number of years greater than the atoms of dust there are in the "hundreds of thousands of myriads of *koti** of the universe." And the assembly of monks thus answers that such an order of magnitude goes "beyond the range of thought."

Expressing what is beyond the range of thought requires words beyond words. For language springs up from the world's flesh. It is deeply embodied in the aspect of beings and in objects visibly revealed. It is as if words shy away when they need to describe the state of mind that realizes voidness, or the inherent absence of existence, of people and phenomena. For voidness, or emptiness, does not mean nothingness. Voidness is the perception of interdependence, of the participative nature of life in which everything is linked. When the mind integrates voidness or emptiness, it can see in an atom as many Buddhas as there are atoms in the universe. Or it perceives the universe in a grain of rice.

A grain of rice is the result of an uninterrupted cosmic process of germination and maturation, unifying the sky, the earth, the elements, and human action, following the rhythm of seasons, which is determined by the revolutions of our planet, the moon, and the sun. A grain of rice makes up a whole, an unfinished, perpetually transforming entity.

In the dimension of voidness, a cloud can also be heard in the bell. How can the cloud be heard through the sound of the bell? If we reconstruct the genesis of the bell, at the beginning there is the

---

* A *koti* is a figure equal to ten million.

cloud, bearing rain. It fertilizes the earth, from which the roots of trees draw water and nutrients for their growth. Then the wood chopped by the woodcutter is set down into a hearth. It feeds the fire of the blacksmith and melts the bronze to cast the bell.

"You have within you the wisdom that heals."

The tiny grain of rice and the immaterial sound of the bell are bearers of immensity. Being aware of the absence of the inherent existence of the grain of rice or of the bell, in other words being in voidness or emptiness, there is no limit to time and space. The wisdom that considers people and phenomena in their primal voidness goes beyond duality. At that point, the world ceases to appear as a collection of independent and separate objects, which illusion differentiates for ordinary consciousness. We understand that all phenomena proceed from the power of the mind and from the natural radiance of wisdom — all phenomena, including those of material, solid, or physical nature. Because they do not have within themselves the causes of their existence, they are therefore empty, as evanescent and stealthy as a rainbow, a mirage, a reflection, or a dream. Contemporary physics confirms this understanding of reality, since the analysis of particles of matter show they are neither indivisible nor permanent. Space is saturated by unsubstantial, impermanent, and unpredictable energies.

"You have within you the wisdom that heals."

From the point of view of ultimate wisdom, my gangrenous leg, my purulent wound, the bone tuberculosis that is breaking my vertebrae, and the pleurisy drowning my lungs are just illusory manifestations. They only have the power to make me suffer if I limit myself to their physical dimension. Admittedly, it is undeniable that I am feeling pain, and if I identify with it, I am reduced to pain, suffering, and agony. Whereas I could transform it into an experience of the mind — a mind that is also empty, unsubstantial, and luminous. My illness is the display of my consciousness, which feels it. If I can perceive it as a pure expression of my mind, and remain within this perception, I will find a space of peace. It will then be possible to liberate the healing energy lying within the subtle levels of the mind.

Maybe I will also have a chance to exhaust a karma of my lineage that expressed itself in the illness affecting the leg of the seventh Phakyab Rinpoche and is being carried on with my gangrene? When such illnesses appear in spiritual masters, they ripen not only their own karma, but also the karma of a great number of beings they are related to. In that sense, they are deeply beneficial.

"You have within you the wisdom that heals."

This illness is a blessing. For the ordinary monk I am, the humble link in an extraordinary lineage of awakened beings, it is an opportunity to purify an overflowing of negative karma that is ripening within me. It is as if the pain that struck me at the very moment I landed on American soil was the sign that old karmas were manifesting, in connection with all of these unknown people, these strangers, who have spontaneously been helping me since my arrival in the United States. The same gangrene, and all the pains that come with it, would not have had the same impact in Tibet or in India. It is undoubtedly what Kundun implies: "Once healed, you will teach the world how to heal." The pain of exile, and of uprooting, will make my healing universal, insofar as I am able to transcend my suffering in the dimension of compassion for all beings, in a prayer that will bathe the world in the spirit of love of Buddhas.

Kundun, My Source of Refuge in This Life and in All My Lives

I am filled with gratitude for the Dalai Lama. This life will not suffice to express to him all of my gratitude. I remember the first time I saw his portrait. One of my uncles was hiding it preciously behind the loose stone of a wall in his house. It was wrapped up in a *katha*, a white, silk scarf of bliss, and protected by a silver reliquary so that mice would not nibble at it. My uncle was risking his life and the security of his family, if unfortunately the Chinese police found that he had kept this picture. On the occasion of family gatherings, and in the secrecy of his home, it was a real ceremony when he showed us this timeworn photograph. It showed Kundun when he was young, wearing big rectangular, horn-rimmed glasses that made his juvenile face look older.

The wooden table on which my uncle would set the portrait was first meticulously cleaned. Then my aunt would cover it with a colored brocade cloth, and she would light a butter lamp. The whole family would murmur the compassion mantra, as we could not chant it aloud for fear of being overheard or denounced. We had no *mala*; they were forbidden, just like all other ritual objects. But the older ones would gently make the familiar gestures of telling their beads between their fingers. The children were also contemplative, and we would softly chant this age-old prayer of the Country of Snow. Calling upon the jewel within the lotus, we could feel the spirit of compassion brushing our lips: *"Om mani padme hum.... Om mani padme hum.... Om mani padme hum...."*

One mantra after another, garlands of mantras coming from our breaths. We visualized them on our hearts, in the clear light of Buddha who cherishes all beings, enlightening the different realms of existence with the radiance of his unconditional love. The reliquary always opened with a sharp snap, and my uncle would pull out Kundun's photo. He laid it down with care onto the square of brocade, and we gazed at it silently, our hands together. My parents and Momola would wipe a few tears, and we would gather our thoughts, united in the compassionate fervor that filled our hearts with joy. It was only with Mao's death, and the liberalization of the 1980s, that portraits of the Dalai Lama reappeared in public. Until they were banished again, banned for fear of prison.

At the age of thirteen, when my parents agreed on my becoming a monk, I was taught the alphabet by the same uncle who kept the photo of the Dalai Lama, and the first text he had me decipher was his Long Life Prayer. I learned it with the Refuges, reciting by heart:

> In this pure land surrounded by the snowy mountains,
> You are the source of all benefit and happiness without
>   exception,
> All powerful Avalokiteshvara, Tenzin Gyatso,
> May you stay immovable until samsara becomes
>   exhausted.

Later on, the links I felt with Kundun guided all the decisive events of my life. In 1985, I wanted to go into exile in India to be closer to him. But I did not dare do it for fear of hurting my grandmother, who loved me so. I had reason to believe that she wouldn't survive my being far away. As my master and other monks were secretly preparing their departure, it was not without some sadness that I gave up the idea of joining them. But, a few days before the date, Momola left her body very peacefully. It was a sign. She was setting me free and blessing me. Before I left, my mother solemnly held me tightly against her, but she bade me farewell without crying. Her constant prayers were with me.

The first time I was blessed by Kundun was in February 1985 in Dharamsala. He held my head between his hands and blew on the top of my skull, fondly calling me "my son." I felt his energy flowing through me, and I was shaking all over. Today, I think that moment, which seemed like a rebirth, was before I was recognized nine years later as the eighth Phakyab Rinpoche.

Being called Kundun's "son" corresponded to the karmic fructification of my merits and of my happy dispositions. I thus started a new life on the path of Awakening. I did not know it at the time, but I understood later that the uncommon intensity of that instant reached the hamlet where I was born. Overwhelmed by a tremendous gratitude toward my mother and the close ones who had helped me grow up, I prayed that the Dalai Lama's blessings would reach out to them — which occurred in the form of a prodigious event.

One fine morning, my mother saw our river as if colored by milk, spotlessly white. Rainbows were floating on the water. It was not a hallucination, since the neighbors also noticed this phenomenon, which became a subject of amazement and endless conversations. My mother said nothing. But in her heart, she felt reassured. To her, it was the undeniable sign that I had not only reached India unharmed, but that I had joined Kundun. When she told me about it, we matched up the dates of this supernatural event and the Dalai Lama's blessing. It was obvious that the dates coincided. I do not interpret this as a miracle, but as the law of *tendrel*, "interdependence." Phenomena, in the physical world, occur according to a causality that is not only material but that also acts from mind to mind. That is because all beings are intimately linked in the network of life. That is why it is important to send out positive thoughts, dedicated to the well-being of all. The love and prayers that we allow to flow from our hearts are extremely powerful. Usually, we cannot objectively verify such occurrences, but on that particular day, my mother in Tibet and I in India were united in Kundun's blessing. The nectar of his compassion became externally visible in the dimension of perception, giving a milky and rainbow aspect to the river of my childhood flowing under Amala's eyes.

The Dalai Lama's Private Office, in charge of welcoming monks who have recently arrived from Tibet, sent me to Sera Mey Monastery in southern India. The Dalai Lama came there regularly to give teachings to the monastic community. Seven years later, in 1992, I received directly from him my vows as a fully ordained monk, and in 1994, he officially recognized me as the eighth Phakyab Rinpoche. I saw him again in an audience in his private apartments in 1997 when he gave me precise instructions to go teach in Tibet. Then, I saw him in 2002, after the hardships of imprisonment in Tibet, and again in 2003, when he urged me to go teach in a Dharma center in the United States. Finally, on November 16, 2003, I sent him my letter, and since November 21, I have been spending many hours meditating each word of his answer, lying in my hospital bed. On all of these occasions, I have blended my mind with his, merging in the space of his boundless compassion.

CHAPTER EIGHT

My Meditation Grotto in Brooklyn

A New Life Is Starting

Monday, December 1, 2003. Under scattered flakes of snow, Pema Dorje comes to pick me up at the hospital. One of his friends has lent him a car. Pema lives in a small apartment in Brooklyn, which, unasked, he has offered to share with me. Till then, I didn't know where I'd go once I left Bellevue Hospital.

Near the Williamsburg Bridge, whose steel cables tighten their clean lines above the East River toward Manhattan, the neighborhood seems to me peaceful and unpretentious. Its rows of well-lined little houses are no more than four or five stories high. The dwellings are sometimes twinned, sometimes separated, edged with tiny landscaped courtyards, looking rather drab and neglected. There is some dullness in the very similar proportions and shapes of the buildings. The only contrast is in the ill-assorted construction materials. In the uniform cityscape we go through, I can see concrete, red bricks, stones, and wood.

Pema Dorje lives on the first floor of a little three-story building, which is rented out by Mr. Lee, a Chinese man in his fifties. There are two rooms separated by an open kitchen and a bathroom. Pema Dorje settles me in his bedroom, which overlooks an inner courtyard. He will occupy the noisier living room over-looking the street. I am deeply moved by his simple and complete generosity, as we enjoy a Tibetan lunch. A new life is starting.

I have no idea what is going to happen to me in the days and weeks to come. Before leaving the hospital, I came up against the care team's lack of understanding of my choice. The doctors were convinced that I would accept amputation. To convince me, they even scheduled meetings with amputees who were relearning how to function after their operation. I am grateful to them for their efforts, and I understood that they interpreted my refusal as a challenge. I had hoped they would let me return to the hospital for regular checkups. This aftercare would have allowed them to examine the evolution of my gangrene. But they answered that, since I had refused the operation, they could do nothing else for me. Even X-rays were not justified outside of treatment. They said they had tried everything they could to save my leg, which was true, and since antibiotic therapy was unsuccessful, the only other option they had was amputation. While one orthopedist lamented that I might soon face an amputation below the hip, oth-ers did not mention this anymore. But I could read that verdict in their eyes.

However, the hospital did impose a medical protocol to treat my tuberculosis, and they did so without asking for my agree-ment. For my application for asylum to have a chance of succeed-ing, this illness had to be eradicated. Because of this, a nurse was scheduled to come visit me in Brooklyn every morning for a shot, and I would go back to the clinic for Survivors of Torture every two months for an X-ray of my lungs and spine.

The nurses who had cleansed and dressed the wound on my ankle every day were sad to see me go. Because of the doctors' very negative prognosis, they felt I would not survive very long.

They prepared for me a supply of compresses (to improve blood circulation), sterile gauze, and plaster. They added a bottle of antiseptics and a local analgesic, and they gave me instructions on how to cleanse my wound. I thanked them, moved by the attention, care, and devotion they had continued to show me.

In Pema Dorje's bedroom, I fill seven copper bowls, which he had placed for me on a shelf, with the water of ritual offerings. Having set up my minimal altar, I forget the hospital. The questions about my illness and my future suddenly fade. My mind becomes absorbed in the present, in the presence of the Buddhas that I call upon. On the first of December, 2003, on the first floor at 265 Manhattan Avenue in Brooklyn, a little room becomes my meditation grotto.

Similar to when I was a child, and I used to call upon the hawk's protection, on this day I call upon my lineage for protection. The spirit of my lineage is not long in manifesting itself, for I perceive a protective, luminous, and benevolent aura — one that reminds me of the bird that unfolded its wings to protect me when, at the age of four, I got lost alone at nightfall in a thunderstorm. Today I am thirty-seven and isolated in New York City, and the threat overhanging me is not a thunderstorm but a serious illness. With the strength of newfound confidence, I grab my bag to pull out the book that has always been with me since my first master in meditation, Geshe Ake Gyupa, gave it to me at Golok Monastery.

I relive the exceptional circumstances of the transmission of this text. It is a bundle of fifty-eight long, rectangular leaves, very tightly enveloped in an orange piece of cloth with a red square sewn on it, held by a string. This *pecha* is the only object I brought with me from Tibet. It is the link between today and my first years of dedicated life, between Brooklyn and Golok Monastery.

How Would You See the Sun outside of You
If You Didn't Have the Sun within You?

The gate at Golok stands at the entrance of a smooth-walled, saffron-colored canyon. These premises are marked by the raw power of the elements, which are displayed in a mandala where terrestrial energy vibrates with an inner fire and is felt in the pure harmonics of a nearby waterfall in the absolute transparence of the air. As a child I fed on the strengths of this miniature cosmos, the intensity of which contains the power of a gestating world. In the months to come, they will help me anchor my meditation in New York City, where I am cut off from natural life and its powers.

The zeal with which, as a child, I imagined jokes and tricks of all sorts was the same energy I channeled as a teenager into my monastic studies and the practice of meditation. My masters were happy to see me making progress. Six months after my arrival at Golok Monastery, I hardly ever left my meditation box. This wooden, ten-square-foot enclosure, which I handcrafted myself, only allowed me to sit cross-legged. I assiduously practiced inner peace meditation, *shamatha*, guided by Geshe Ake Gyupa.

Of great stature, Geshe-la was an old man with a dry, bony face. His eyes seemed huge. I have never, in any landscape, gazed at an abyss as deep as his look. I worshipped him tremendously, and I would toe the line with him. Seeing my progress in developing mental peace, he offered to teach me practices that only experienced meditators are entitled to.

Geshe-la introduced me to the *tsa-lung*, a Tibetan word meaning "wind channels," by initiating me to the Mandala of Chakrasamvara, a tantric deity whose meditation stirs up the fire of primal wisdom. Known as the "Wheel of Great Bliss," this meditation belongs to the collection of mother tantras that, like all of Buddha's teachings, are based on the four noble truths. The first noble truth is that the suffering of all beings is the result of conditioned existence. The second one is understanding the causes of this suffering. The third one is the cessation of all suffering by implementing a method, and the fourth one is following the path to be delivered from suffering, the state of Awakening. The Chakrasamvara Yoga systems lead to freedom from suffering by purifying the energy, and the psychophysical components of the body, thanks to visualizing tantric deities, and their attributes, in their perfectly pure environment, the mandala. These deities are not outside the meditator. They symbolize different dimensions of one's mind-body continuum: "There are several bodies within your body," Geshe Ake Gyupa often said.

Geshe-la smiled at me whenever he saw me touching my arms or my hands as if to convince myself of their reality. He would say: "Your hands, your arms, your eyes, your ears, your teeth, your bones, your flesh are not you. No more than your blood, your muscles, or your organs are the essence of who you are. Your physical body, as you can see it, touch it, or feel it, is not your only body. Within the limits of your physical shape, there is an intangible, conscious body, linked with deep levels of your mind. Meditation consists in identifying these more and more subtle levels to understand who you really are and who you can become. As you go, you will experience a wisdom and a bliss you cannot even fathom right now."

Geshe-la's words were not abstract; as he spoke, he would demonstrate simple but deep breathing exercises. By associating them with the concentration I had developed with *shamatha*, little by little I was able to identify the flows of energy in my body. Today, I am infinitely grateful to him for adapting these precious teachings to my level as a beginner. He would explain: "The sun you can see shining in the sky is also within you. In you, it does not appear as the star that warms you by day. In you, it is the energy of fire flowing through your subtle channel on the right. This energy regulates bilious humor and the negative emotions of anger, hatred, and aversion. Transformed, sublimated, this inner sun becomes the awakened wisdom of space that is embodied by the dakinis."

Geshe-la would ask me to first visualize my energetic body as an empty enclosure, a shallow shell of light — without flesh, without bones, without muscles — with three main channels along the axis of my spine. The central channel is bright, thin, and red on the inside and lapis lazuli blue on the outside. The lateral channels, envisioned with the same finesse and transparency, are red on the right and white on the left.

Geshe-la would explain to me how to follow the movement of my breath, inhaling through the right nostril with a gesture of the hand, while blocking the left nostril, then making air descend to the root of one's breath, four fingers below the navel, where the hands of Buddhas are placed during meditation. Then I would bring up the toxins of the right channel and breathe them out through the left nostril.

"Just as the sun is within you, the moon is, too. Learn how to recognize it. It flows in the shape of water and earth energy, in your subtle channel on the left."

Then I would open the left channel to let the lunar energy flow out and eliminate the negativities of phlegmatic humor and the associated feelings of desire and attachment. In full consciousness, I would inhale air through the left nostril, visualizing it as a river of light, and then breathe it out on the right. I learned to concentrate my attention on the movements of energy in the central channel, which corresponds, on an external level, to the eclipse of the sun and the moon. Breathing with both nostrils, I would maximize the potential of air energy in relation to wind humor and the emotion of ignorance.

Following Geshe-la's instructions, I applied myself to discovering the universe following the rhythm of my breath. Such a close, deep, and vibrating universe! I would direct all of my energies toward the inside. I would swallow infinity! I would breathe immensity! It was altogether familiar and different from the sensations of boundlessness that had filled my childhood on the high plateaus. Then, my mind was still living in the external and physical envelope of the world. Now, I was discovering inner space without beginning or end. Geshe-la said:

Remember that these breathing practices are not only physical. You are not just breathing with your lungs. You are not just breathing oxygen. When you inhale air, undoubtedly you need this air to renew the cells of your blood. But just as your body has a subtle and hidden aspect, breathing also has a subtle counterpart. The *lung*, or "winds," make life force move around, also called *prana*, an energy that brings to life all sentient beings, as well as planets and celestial bodies. Life force irrigates all the channels, starting with the navel chakra, where there are twelve channels corresponding to the twelve astrological houses, divided into two types of energy, lunar and solar.

From the right nostril, it is the solar winds that flow, and from the left one, the lunar winds. They magnetize the 360 winds corresponding to the 360 days of the lunar calendar, and they circulate in the channels of the wheel at the navel. These 360 winds are coupled with the winds of the elements: earth, water, fire, air, and space. If the winds in one day are multiplied by the winds of the elements, the result is a total of 1,800 winds, half of which are solar, and the other half lunar. As there are twelve "great winds" within the twenty-four hours of a day, it comes to 21,600 winds. Combined with the elements, these winds

transit through the different chakras and give them energy. Thus, the earth wind activates the corresponding
chakra at the navel; the water wind activates the correlate
heart chakra; for the fire wind, it is the throat chakra; and
for the air wind, the crown chakra.

Geshe-la passed on to me the essence of his wisdom, born
in the heart of his experience as a yogi, in this life and in his past
lives. I dove joyfully into the ocean of his mind. He made me understand that the alternation of day and night is also an inner phenomenon.

"How would you see the sun outside of you if you didn't have
the sun within you? The moon outside of you if you didn't have
it inside you?" Geshe-la asked me one day, bursting into an infectious uncontrollable laughter.

That is how I experienced inexpressible daybreaks, supreme
full moon risings, and inner eclipses with diamond crowns. The
sky was my mind. I was the sky.

Later on, seeing pictures of the moon taken by astronauts,
this heavenly body would look oddly dead to me. It was like the
carcass of a moon compared to the moon living within me. In
fact, some lamas had a hard time believing this happened. A man
walked on the moon in 1969?

"Which moon?" Geshe-la would ask.

The moon of his meditations seemed to him much more real
than the one on which Neil Armstrong planted the starry banner
of the United States. He said, "The real conquest of space is of
the inner space that contains all worlds. Any other conquest, of a
material nature, is an illusion."

To conquer this inner space, Geshe-la advised me to cultivate the breathing yoga practices, starting with the "nine cycles,"
which are based on the movements of in-breath, out-breath, and
retention, and which correlate to the three subtle channels on the

right, left, and middle. This is also called the "practice of the three vacuities," since visualizing the empty body, the empty channels, and the empty chakras is associated with these breathings. The channels do not intersect like in an ordinary state, where they form the knots of the chakras, the "psychophysical centers" of the subtle body. The energies circulate without being obstructed along rectilinear channels. They are thus able to liberate obstructions that deviate or limit the flow of energy. This results in restoring the balance of the elements, on a subtle level, while restoring harmony in the three humors, on a physical level, which guarantees good health.

Healing Sciences and Inner Yoga Practices

There is a very fine anatomy of the subtle body. Geshe-la taught this to me with the help of painted plates created by an artist monk, Lobsang Woeser, who followed Geshe-la's instructions very closely. However, Geshe-la reminded me constantly: "What you can see here on these pictures has no more reality than the rainbow or the reflection of the moon on water."

I memorized the names of the chakras, which we called wheels in *tsa-lung* meditations, or lotuses in deity yoga practices. They are lined up along the central axis of the body. Geshe-la explained: "The central channel is also called the 'channel of secrecy,' for its essence goes beyond words. Its essence is Awakening. But Awakening cannot be told. It is experienced. Imagine the central channel as a ray of sunshine. It goes down to the secret organ, and its tip opens up at the crown chakra of your head. This point is called the 'Door to Brahma,' for that is where consciousness is ejected at death to go to the pure lands. The central channel is like a stem going through the center of all the root chakras. Thus it is compared to the axle of the wheel of chakras."

Along the central channel, which runs parallel to the spine,

I learned to identify the five root chakras that are the "main wheels." On the head, the "Wheel of Great Bliss" has sixteen spokes and is reflected in the "ocean of nerves" of the brain. This chakra is green and associated with the wind element. At the base of the throat, the "Wheel of Perfect Enjoyment" has thirty-two spokes, is red, and is associated with fire. It is called the "gateway to dreams," for that is where the mind dwells when we fall asleep. At the heart, the white "Wheel of Reality," has eight spokes, is associated with water, and is the basis of consciousness. The heart chakra is also called the "Wheel of Phenomena." Its eight spokes correspond to the eight states of consciousness: five states of sensory consciousness, plus mental consciousness, emotional consciousness, and all-encompassing foundation consciousness. At the navel, the yellow "Wheel of Emanation" has sixty-four spokes and is the seat of the Earth. It is the chakra that tsa-lung practices work from. At the secret organ, the "Wheel of the Pres- ervation of Bliss" has thirty-two spokes, and its blue color corre- sponds to the space element.

I also learned to count the secondary chakras: These are in the joints of the upper limbs in the shoulders, the elbows, and the wrists; in the lower limbs at the hips, the knees, and the ankles; and in the phalanxes of the fingers and the toes.

There are many other channels, too many for artists to re- produce. They all form the network of the 72,000 channels of a perfect human body, to which the tantras add 14,400,000 tiny channels corresponding to the skin pores and to the hairs. In ico- nography, they appear in the form of thin lines in gold paint that artists draw radiating around awakened beings.

The subtle anatomy is the vajra body, which is translated as "adamantine body," since diamonds have the reputation of being unbreakable. In the same way, the channels, contrary to their bodily counterparts, are indestructible, for they are animated by the life of the mind, which is pure light.

Geshe Ake Gyupa taught me:

Recognizing the true nature of the mind, such is the ultimate goal of breathing yoga, the basis of which I have given you, and that you will go deeper into. You will achieve that by bringing the winds of sun and moon into the central channel. When, during your meditation, these two stars reach a state of conjunction, like the eclipses that we can see in the sky, you will reach the state of union. The merging of the feminine winds, of solar nature, with the masculine winds, of lunar nature, is shown in sacred art by the coupling of the father and mother deities. Their embrace symbolizes the experience of fulfillment. It can be felt as a blissful vibration, and it leads to the disappearance of distressing emotions, these veils that cast a shadow on the mind. In this state of divine union, all appearances will become pure bliss, and you will experience the breath of clear light.

Geshe-la described to me the state of meditative contemplation that one can reach at that stage, when the five eyes open: the physical eye, the eye of wisdom, the divine eye, the eye of Dharma, and the eye of Buddha. The yogi then experiences extrasensory powers that allow for miraculous accomplishments, like being able to hear or see with no notion of distance, to read the thoughts of others, and to remember one's former lives through all the trichiliocosm, or the billion-fold universe of Buddhist cosmology.

"Such are the unconceivable fruits of completely mastering the winds and the mind," Geshe-la asserted.

He told me all this with perfect modesty, without trying to impress me. I had tremendous affection for him as he guided me with natural authority, without severity, and through experience, so that I could also follow the path of realization that leads to Awakening. Of the many methods he taught me, I can say nothing. Neither can I tell about the results or the signs of success I experienced. Some day, I hope to be able to share all of this with students whom I have specially prepared to receive such knowledge.

According to tradition, these teachings are to be kept under the seal of secrecy, which I have never contravened. The aim of such secrecy is not to save this knowledge for a few privileged people. The secret is the secret of experience. Words alone are incapable of translating these experiences, and if someone tried, the words might be misleading. Without the precise instructions of a master who has himself traveled this path of deep wisdom, minds that are unstable — that have not been trained, prepared, and calmed beforehand — would risk being unable to distinguish their own mental disruptions. They might take their hallucinations for the genuine experience of the central channel, and these practices could, in the end, turn out to be dangerous.

The Body Does Not Heal Thanks to the Body.
The Body Heals Thanks to the Mind.

With benevolence, Geshe Ake Gyupa warned me against false interpretations that would be detrimental to my practice. He insisted on one particular point: "*Tsa* is translated as 'channel,' but don't forget that, literally, this word means 'root.' A root, under the earth, is invisible. But that is what transforms the energy of Mother Earth into nourishing sap. In the same way, in our body, the channels remain invisible. They don't appear in the same way as blood vessels, nerves, or tendons do because they are as immaterial in essence as the mind. Yet it is in these subtle channels that the body draws its energy and that life flows. Only clairvoyant beings who have developed inner vision can see the network of channels lighting up the inside of the physical body. The earth of the channels is your mind. You can give them life and control them in meditation through the mind."

During the weeks before I moved into Pema Dorje's apartment, I unceasingly recollected Geshe Ake Gyupa's instructions. He once said something that, in my present situation, seems prescient: "When you reach an advanced level of inner energy yoga practice, you will be able to reconstruct channels that have been cut or damaged in your body. Your practice of energy yoga in the channels will help you repair your physical body. The body does not heal thanks to the body. The body heals thanks to the mind."

As I remembered this, the path to my recovery opened. I knew I had to follow the teachings that I once received at Golok Monastery.

"You have within you the wisdom that heals," Kundun said in his message.

The Dalai Lama knows I have been trained in the *tsa-lung* inner sciences and yoga practices. I told him about it. He thought I had been very lucky to receive such teachings from a genuine master who had experienced them himself in all their depth. Nowadays, more than before, one runs the risk of being trained by people whose minds have not matured enough through experience. Their understanding remains mainly intellectual. But intellectually, only the peel of the practice can be understood. The fruit is not given to us. If the fruit has not yet matured in the master's consciousness, how can it appear in the disciple? The dimension of inner transformation is lacking, and this is the only way to make direct transmission, from mind to mind, possible.

The Mind Is the Best Doctor, the Best Remedy

I gently pull on the string around the *pecha* that Geshe Ake Gyupa gave me at Golok Monastery not long before he left his body. I recall his words: "I have given you the transmission of *tsa-lung*, which is ordinarily only for advanced meditators. I felt your stream of consciousness was mature enough to receive it. Take this *pecha* in which you will find my practice notes. You will perfectly understand them later on in relation to the teachings I have given you. My notes should help you make progress on your own path of experience. You have the potential to become an accomplished *tsa-lung* practitioner."

At the time, I protested, asking Geshe-la to offer this book to another, older, and more advanced disciple who would make better use of it.

"It is not up to you to judge that!"

Such was the brief answer he gave me. There was no answering back.

Without contradicting my master any longer, I prostrated myself before him. He made me promise I would never open this book in front of anyone: "Nobody must take a look at this manuscript. It contains the essence of my practice of *tsa-lung*. I am transmitting it to you. To you. To you only. This book is alive. You will need it some day, and you will consult it as if you were consulting a benevolent friend. And on that day, its pages will speak to you and will tell you what no human being could ever tell you. It will be infinitely precious. In such moments, I will be with you in mind, as close as we have been in these last three years. Our destinies are going to part, but our consciousnesses will remain united in the luminous basis of awakened wisdom."

Geshe Ake Gyupa held my face between his hands and put his forehead for a long time on mine. Heartbroken, I felt this moment was a farewell. We never saw each other again.

The foretold day has arrived. It is today, December 1, 2003. My last meeting with Geshe-la was exactly twenty years ago. I carefully unfold the fabric around his *pecha*. I suddenly interrupt my movements. With my eyes closed, I become impregnated with the incense fragrance rising from the book. I recognize a sandal-wood smell that was very dear to my master. Moved to tears, I can feel his presence. Just as he had predicted, he is back with me when I need him. He is here. His mind is here in my mind.

With infinite respect, with tremendous gratitude, I turn the leaves. As I turn the pages, his fine handwriting takes off, and the Tibetan cursive gives it an aspect of musical staves. As if the book, before speaking to me, were whispering to me a song, a song of trust, of trust in Geshe-la's word, of trust in his promise, which is being fulfilled. Carried away by this trust where there is no place for doubt, I can hear him telling me: "The mind is the best doctor. The mind is the best remedy."

With these words, I recover a serenity I have not felt in a long time, since my arrival in New York City, six months ago.

Through Prayer, I Was United to All Beings

I determine the program of my practices, which will not change until my full recovery three years later in December 2006. My typ-ical day starts at five o'clock in the morning. I first chant prayers of refuge and tribute to Je Tsongkhapa, then to my lineage. After that, I arrange the offerings to the Buddhas and recite the prayers of *bodhicitta*, the spirit of altruistic Awakening, until six o'clock. That is when Pema Dorje leaves to go to work. Meanwhile, I start my practice of *tsa-lung*, which lasts one hour. I meditate the Med-icine Buddha and *tong-len*, universal compassion, and I chant the mantras of Hayagriva, a wrathful expression of the Buddha of Compassion.

A horse-headed deity with a human body, Hayagriva has the power to assist beings in the six realms of existence. His body is red, and his flaming hair is bristling, while an eye of transcendent wisdom cuts the middle of his forehead. His four hands brandish a lasso and an ax, which are intended for capturing and destroying the demons and obstacles that distress sick people, whose suffering is provoked by wicked spirits. I therefore chant for an hour the invocation to Hayagriva, which sounds like the neighing of a horse.

At nine o'clock, I pause for breakfast.

At ten, I go back to my room. A new session starts with the master's yoga, a contemplative practice of Yamantaka, one of the main deities of Je Tsongkhapa and of the lamas of my lineage. A wrathful expression of Manjushri, Yamantaka, in his very angry appearance, embodies awakened wisdom. His name in Sanskrit means "conqueror of death," since Yamantaka eradicates ignorance, which is the cause of dualism or the fragmented appearance of reality. In this ferocious aspect, the wisdom of emptiness returns to the world, grounding it in primordial, luminous, and loving purity, without beginning or end, without birth or death. This state beyond ignorance and illusion, with its trail of emotions and attachment, is embodied by Yamantaka, who has nine faces, thirty-four arms, and sixteen legs. His main head is that of a buffalo and is surmounted by Manjushri. His dark blue body bears the color of emptiness. His bone jewels, his crown of fifty-one freshly severed heads, and the knife of the dakinis, which he brandishes while making the terrifying *mudra* threat with his hand, symbolize the action of wisdom dismembering the body of dualistic illusions, wringing their neck, and stripping them to the bone. This meditation, in which I unite my mind with the energy of primordial wisdom, is a strong antidote to obstacles and illness.

"When you meditate on a deity," Geshe Ake Gyupa instructed me, "never forget that it has no material appearance, no external existence. The deity that you visualize with a body, clothes, jewels, and attributes belongs to your inner mandala. It is none other than your own mind appearing to you in this shape.

By remembering that there is no difference between the deity and your own root lama, you will be in that very moment linked with the empty nature of clear light, the essence of the deity, the essence of your guru, the essence of the gurus of your lineage and of yourself. You will then be revealed your loving and luminous basis of wisdom."

In Tibet we say that, just as a bird cannot fly without both its wings, the mind needs the wings of wisdom and compassion to be able to spread. That is why, after having contemplated wisdom in its pure state in the manifested shapes of Hayagriva and of Yamantaka, I call upon Green Tara. Born from a tear of compassion shed by Avalokiteshvara when faced with the inexhaustible pains of the world, she embodies the feminine side of compassion of all Buddhas and the essence of their awakened activity. Her green color, symbolizing the air element, whose purified aspect she embodies, is associated with the movement of thoughts. She helps those who meditate with the swiftness of wind. She is the original Tara, and the twenty-one Taras I offer my praises to are aspects of her. *Tara* means "she who rescues," as well as "star," for she shines in the night of our suffering to guide us on the path to liberation. The feminine power of compassion embodied by Tara links us to the deepest energies of transformation, protection, and healing of the mind. Her practice transforms negative into positive, at the most subtle level of our continuum of consciousness and of the events affecting us. Tara is called the "mother of all Buddhas," since meditating on her develops unconditional love and compassion, which are the basis of Awakening for all beings.

I continue my prayers for Tara by chanting her mantra, and then I proceed with an accumulation of Medicine Buddha mantras until 1 PM. After a simple and frugal lunch, generally based on roasted barley flour and cheese, I resume chanting Medicine Buddha mantras around 3 PM. Bearing the color of the lapis lazuli medicinal stone, Sangye Menla, the Medicine Buddha, embodies the ultimate healing that occurs upon realizing the awakened essence of the mind. Calling upon him gives access to the innate healing powers of the natural world, which are found in the consciousness of any living being. During this three-year retreat, I will chant two hundred *malas* to Sangye Menla every day, meaning that each day I chant his mantra twenty thousand times.

At 6 PM, I drink a warm cup of tea and carry on accumulating mantras until Pema Dorje comes back around 8 PM. We share supper, and I help him clear the table and put the dishes away. Then I meditate for at least two hours, before ending with my dedication of merits to all beings and prayers of long life to Kundun. I never go to bed before midnight.

Some dates in the lunar month are dedicated to Tara, to the Medicine Buddha, to Amitabha, to Padmasambhava, to the dakinis, and to invoking protectors. On those days, I more particularly intensify their specific practices, accompanying them with lengthy offerings of the universe mandala. But I keep up the daily *tsa-lung*, Green Tara, and Medicine Buddha meditations. I occasionally have to shorten my practices during the day because of a medical appointment. I then stay up later to finish my mantra recitations.

In retrospect, I would say that during those three years, the days went by one after the other without my ever becoming bored by the repetition of practices. It never became monotonous. It was as if, during each session, I were becoming another, renewing myself in the outpouring of wisdom and compassion that springs from meditation. Every day was a gratifying day.

The essence of my practice was based on the awareness that everything is linked. Nothing exists independently, contrary to the ordinary perception of reality, which conceives of a self that is isolated from the whole, a self that is wrongly perceived as autonomous. This idea distinguishes, divides, and separates people and world phenomena, causing attachment, aversion, hatred, anger, and frustration. The texture of these negative emotions gives birth to illusions, which are believed to be realities. These illusions are the cause of deep sufferings and unpleasant experiences, which are corrupted by self-cherishing. The extreme duality between self and the rest of the world destroys our natural peace of mind. This duality is the origin of all the conflicts we experience, on an individual and on a global scale.

My masters taught me: "All the sufferings come from the mind; we can erase them with the mind. They will disappear like the rainbow, without trace. By developing *bodhicitta*, the heart of Awakening that cherishes others more than oneself, you will dispel your suffering and that of others. Sublime wisdom, which protects from suffering, will emerge within you."

Throughout those days of solitary retreat, I thus applied myself to contemplating the wisdom that understands the interdependency of everything. I lived with that awareness every second of every day, enlightened by the spirit of love and compassion of the Buddhas. Love and compassion are two aspects of the same feeling of benevolence. Love is wishing all beings might be happy and seeking to bring together the causes for their happiness. Compassion is wishing that they might be freed from suffering, and I offered my prayers to create the merits that would empty the samsara of all forms of suffering.

By meditating love and compassion, I developed the spontaneous feeling of being linked to all lives. As I continued, experiencing this link through the hardship of illness gave me renewed strength. And I found, by dedicating myself to the well-being of others, the basis of my inner peace. Retired for three years, and solitary, I was alone. And I was not alone. Through prayer, I was united to all beings.

Final Healing

At the age of thirty-seven, I have not been spared the hardships of life. These hardships have been my guru. They have taught me that suffering is natural, that it is part of the wheel of lives. We have been suffering since a time without beginning. Recognizing this suffering is the first noble truth Shakyamuni Buddha founded his teaching on, 2,500 years ago in India. It is not by avoiding suffering that we put an end to it. By understanding it, and accepting it, we stop opposing it, and we have a chance of eliminating it, for ourselves and for all beings.

Accepted suffering is no longer painful. It becomes strength, a power that transforms. For three years, the fire of suffering burned very old karmas within me. In my purified heart, I welcomed the pains of human suffering, and I gave humanity as an offering all the light, all the bliss that was being born within me through practice. I have adopted these recommendations by the yogi Langri Tangpa:

> In brief, may I offer benefit and joy,
> To all my mothers, both directly and indirectly.
> May I quietly take upon myself
> All hurts and pains of my mothers.
> May all this remain undefiled
> By the stains of the eight mundane concerns;*
> And may I, recognizing all things as illusion,
> Devoid of clinging, be released from bondage.

To take upon myself the suffering of beings, and to offer them my happiness, I put into practice the great Indian saint Atisha's

---

* The eight mundane or worldly concerns are hope for happiness and fear of suffering; hope for gain and fear of loss; hope for fame and fear of insignificance; and hope for praise and fear of blame.

advice from the heart. At the beginning of the eleventh century, he came to Tibet to teach the magnificent practices of *tong-len*, the transmission of which I received several times throughout my monastic studies. *Tong-len*, or "taking-giving," is a training of the mind that quickly becomes second nature, for it is associated with a movement that is the source of life: breathing. On the in-breath, we unconditionally welcome all the pains of the six realms of existence. These enter us as black smoke that, without resistance, we allow to flow toward the heart chakra. At the very moment the smoke touches the center of our being, our energy of compassion transforms this energy of suffering. The smoke becomes light. The pain becomes bliss. And we breathe out this bliss, and we completely offer, without reservation, our happiness, and the causes of our happiness, to all beings.

"Don't be afraid of absorbing within you the past, present, and future sufferings of beings," Geshe Ake Gyupa would say to me. "These sufferings, once absorbed in your heart, will be transformed into nectars of bliss. With some training, *tong-len* will become as natural to you as breathing. It will be the sign that you have perfectly integrated the practice."

Day after day, breath after breath, I discover the power of compassion. It is the inexhaustible source of life, for compassion is the nature of Buddha. Only the energy of compassion can bring the paranoia of the ego to an end and stabilize the mind by bringing the hallucinated perceptions of reality to a close. In this sense, compassion is a healing energy, since it purifies the mental poisons and thus makes it possible to access the subtle levels of the mind. In my practices, *tong-len* shows me, more and more clearly, the secret light radiating from the heart.

Geshe-la said: "In the center of the heart chakra shines the mind, which is the essential drop, free from elaboration. It is a luminous sphere, the size of a lentil. It contains the coemerging original wisdom. Its essence is voidness, and its nature nonobstructed clarity."

These teachings of Geshe Ake Gyupa's take on new meaning. They are embodied, lit by compassion. Twenty years later, they are fulfilled. *Tong-len* allows me to deepen the inner yoga energy practices.

On a deep and subtle level, the *tsa-lung* methods regenerate the life-supporting drops or essences, which are called *tigle* in Tibetan, in particular the one that has its seat in the heart. By concentrating on channels and winds, one drives the life force, the *prana*, from the lateral channels to the central channel, since the left and right channels are filled with veiling emotions and with their karmic imprints. Whereas the central channel, called the "mother channel of realization," is by essence nondualistic, like the awakened mind. Endowed with an energy similar to that of a black hole, it absorbs karmic winds and neutralizes them, transforming them into wisdom winds.

"Concentrate intensely on the heart," Geshe Ake Gyupa would say to me. "Focus on the energy that comes out of it. Put your consciousness onto its inner vibration. Just like a mirror that reflects everything without grasping anything, reflect the clear light, and remain without capturing it when it comes to you. In that way, you will awaken to *bodhicitta*, the 'Awakened Mind,' linked with the heart wind uniting felicity and emptiness."

The essence of *tong-len*, as with *tsa-lung*, is the ultimate healing of Awakening. What I have shared of Geshe-la's teachings is only the introduction to the practice. As I've mentioned, regarding the visions I received, the obstacles and how I overcame them, and about the signs and the accomplishments that marked this period — about all that, I am allowed to say nothing. My vows as a monk require me to remain silent.

I See the First Signs of Improvement

Though I am not allowed to disclose my spiritual realizations, I can speak about my physical recovery and about the improvement of my health.

In December, after settling at Pema Dorje's, and contrary to the doctors' repeated assertions that my leg is dead, I continue to feel a sign of life — even if the flesh on my foot has a deathly aspect. The sign is faint but persistent, barely perceptible, like the tiny tip of a delicate green shoot when it springs out of a thunderstruck tree. For, under the ashes of charred bark, tree sap still bears the message of life. I therefore concentrate on the tiny trace of light in my gangrenous ankle. I continuously radiate toward this point the energies of my practices.

I understand quite well that I am doomed by their diagnosis. I understand that the blood flow is obstructed. As a result of not being nourished, the cells cannot regenerate. I undertake to reconstruct the dried-out vessels. To revitalize my physical body, I first have to work on a subtle level. My first efforts thus aim at reactivating the chakra at my ankle joint and at making my life force, the *prana*, flow inside its channels. I devote a part of each practice session to that, as well as to *tsa-lung*.

In the first few weeks, the wound remains putrid and continues weeping. I cleanse it every morning, but I am not able to do a deep curetting in the same way as the nurses at the hospital. I merely remove the fragments of bone carried by the pus and apply warm gauzes to enable vascularization. It does not take long before I see the first signs of improvement. However, then I face the reluctance of the doctors to admit I am getting better. They only acknowledge this once it becomes obvious and impossible to deny — without ever showing interest in the means I am implementing to heal.

The Hospital Reports

In order to treat my tuberculosis, I continue having regular appointments at Bellevue Hospital. On January 21, 2004 — seven weeks after I left the hospital and undertook my own healing retreat — I consult with Dr. Ryan. Since I arrived at Bellevue and joined the Program for Survivors of Torture, this young doctor from New York University has followed my case. He is undoubtedly the most benevolent of all the specialists I have had the privilege to meet. I inform him that the wounds on my ankle are weeping less. He examines me, and indeed, he notices an improvement. Intrigued by this evolution of my gangrene — which he is not expecting — he prescribes an X-ray.

The interpretation of the photo in the radiologist's report is explicit: "A destructive arthritis of the right ankle joint is again noted. Lucency and the periostitis in the region of the right medial malleolus appears to have healed somewhat since the previous study. Moreover, the overall bone density appears more uniform, and there has been interval resolution of some of the mottled osteopenia noted on the earlier examination. The degree of fragmentation and collapse at the articular margins of the right ankle joint — more severe in the talar dome — is essentially unchanged, however. Based on the lateral projections, a right ankle joint effusion is suspected. Mild generalized soft tissue swelling is unchanged."

Dr. Ryan checks my enthusiasm. Remissions sometimes occur, but it does not mean recovery.

"Let's remain careful!" he concludes. "It is extraordinary enough to see that your case has not gotten worse and that we can note some betterment. But the periosteum, the tissue recovering the surface of the bone, is still in an inflammatory state, and unfortunately the diagnosis of septic arthritis is still topical."

However, as the days go by, the process of putrefaction shows very clear signs of regression. It reaches the point where I do not even need to cleanse the wound, and I can see it starting to form a scar. At the same time, my pain is lessening, even when walking, and I can now cross the apartment without crutches. I still need them, of course, to move around in the neighborhood and when I go to the hospital. I hesitate to tell the doctors about this improvement, since they will question it. I also understand that gloating is not welcome.

On July 7, 2004, one of the doctors who had strongly recommended amputation last fall is amazed to see me set my foot on the floor. She notes in her report that there is a very favorable evolution of my gangrene, and that I am not suffering anymore. She asks me what treatment I have been following. I answer that I meditate twelve hours a day. She stares at me, amused. Incredulously, she sighs: "If only one could heal through meditation!"

I am surprised she does not wonder about this more. She sentenced me less than a year ago, claiming that my necrotized leg was dead. Eight months later, she can see it coming back to life. How am I not, in her eyes, a living example of healing through meditation? Originally, she had refused to offer me any other form of treatment aside from amputation, and she even went so far as to be doubtful, aloud, in front of me, that I could survive without it. On that day, I sincerely regretted such terrible lack of understanding.

At regular intervals, I see the same doctor, a pneumonologist who is treating my tuberculosis. We meet on September 29 and on December 29, 2004, and each time, she examines my leg and notes more extensive improvement. On February 16, 2005, she records a new fact that demonstrates unequivocally the progress I am making each week. For now I can walk three blocks without crutches before I need to use them again to ease the pain. I have been testing my strength to see the number of blocks I can walk, following the straight avenue alongside Pema Dorje's apartment. I was hesitant at first; for some weeks I brought both crutches with me in case of weakness. Now, as my confidence increases, I only take one. I do this exercise daily during the lunch break of my retreat. It is encouraging and a source of pride, to be able to overcome gangrene only through meditation.

On September 6, 2005, I declare to this doctor that I can now walk five blocks and stand for two hours without suffering. She notices that the wound has actually formed a scar and that I am recovering the mobility of my ankle. Over two months later, on December 27, she prescribes me a stabilizing ankle-foot orthosis. This light, translucent plastic splint holds and stabilizes the leg, ankle, and foot. This equipment increases my comfort when walking and, above all, prevents me from spraining my ankle. Considering my ankle's weakness, there is always the danger of slipping on it. I use the brace for several months.

Step by step, I recover my strength. When meditating, I still visualize the chakra and the channels of my ankle, which are becoming more and more clear and luminous as they regenerate the structure of my veins and blood vessels. I also encompass all sick people, disabled, and handicapped, taking their pains upon myself and radiating toward them my winds of healing. When I take the subway to go to the hospital, each time I see the homeless — who drive other passengers away because of their repulsive body odors — I feel a surge of deep compassion and draw near them. I have experienced the disgust of purulent flesh and suffered the putrid fumes of my gangrene. How is it possible to believe that they too are not indisposed by their own stench? I can't speak their language, but I spend time near them and visualize them in the blessed light of Buddhas, wrapping their suffering within my silent prayer.

In each car of the subway, I assess all the suffering, the tears, and the despair that I meet. During my monastic training, I encountered lack of food and hygiene, illness, and bereavement. But it has taken my American exile, and the ordeal of gangrene, for me to glimpse the ocean of sufferings in the world. As life flows again in my leg, the Love Sutra prayer spontaneously springs up from my heart with increasing compassion as I witness the visible and invisible despair all around me:

> Just as a mother would protect her only child at the risk
>   of her own life,
> Even so, let us cultivate a boundless heart toward all
>   beings.
> Let our thoughts of boundless loving kindness pervade
>   the whole world,
> Above, below, and across, without obstruction, without
>   any hatred, without any enmity.

The Mind Was Never Born, the Mind Has Never Died

The Experience of Suffering Is Necessary

Ever since the fall of 2006, I have walked normally. I have completely recovered from my gangrene, from my bone tuberculosis, and from my pleurisy. My healing retreat lasted three years.

During those three years, it was thanks to the Dalai Lama's blessing, and by reconnecting with the experience built up during previous lives, that I found the strength to meditate and fully recover. At times, physical pain was more and less severe, but it was rarely absent. Yet I managed to dissociate my mind from these painful feelings. As I was suffering, my mind meditated on emptiness. I imagined that all beings were suffering, too, and just like me, they ardently wanted liberation from their suffering. In these moments, united to all forms of life, in all realms of existence, I experienced the true nature of reality — on two levels of consciousness.

On a relative level, being aware of physical pain anchored me to the first level of reality, that of conditioned existence, which is suffering. On an ultimate level, being aware of peace, joy, and serenity anchored me to the second level of reality, that of compassion. The two coexisted, and they were wiped out when meditating on emptiness. If only people affected by illness, and by the different hardships of existence, could understand how necessary it is to experience pain! We should not flee from it, for fear of maintaining the illusion that all is well and that we can continue as we are. We then lose the basis of our spiritual path, which is accepting that the nature of the body and of life is to suffer. When we are willingly penetrated by this obvious fact, illness becomes a gift. Even bedridden, confined, disabled, or crippled, we can work for the well-being of all and give meaning to omnipresent suffering.

In recovering from my gangrene, I purified a specific karma of my lineage, since the previous Phakyab Rinpoche had suffered from a similar health problem that was carried on in my present incarnation. My illness erupted just as I landed in the West. Then, though I healed in the West, it was outside of the Western health care system. I recovered my health through meditation and inner energy yoga practices. I cannot publicly disclose their essence, but I have vowed to share the practices of *tsa-lung* that cured me with meditators who are sufficiently committed and advanced.

My healing required that I first dispel an illusion — that Western medicine is the panacea — and I have since sought to understand what modern medicine is lacking so badly. At the time, I couldn't grasp how the medical care teams could abandon their vocation — one dedicated to the service of life — by insisting that mutilating surgery was my only choice. In refusing amputation, and in leaving Bellevue Hospital, I had to acknowledge that their medical protocol did not apply to my case. I decided to trust my self-healing capacities, which rested in my practices and training in *tsa-lung*. Without these assets, I do not believe that the Dalai Lama would have invited me to seek healing within. And I believe I would have had the wisdom to agree to the operation I was pressed to accept.

On the other hand, afterward, why did these same doctors,

who had wanted to amputate me, choose to deny my healing? That I cannot understand. They saw the wounds of my gangrene healing, and how I progressively managed to walk without crutches, yet they preferred to ignore what this meant. Was it because it contradicted their disastrous prognosis? Or because I had used the healing potential of the mind?

I have never allowed myself to argue with the doctors over their irreversible necrosis diagnosis, nor over their recommendation to amputate, which they unanimously advised. I have always thanked them for their efforts and expressed to them my sincere gratitude. Conversely, was it too unbearable for them to inquire about my method for healing? Couldn't they have acknowledged having something to learn about healing from a source other than medical school?

I believe the doctors who treated me were and are entirely devoted to the service of their patients. I have not a single doubt that they implement everything they can to cure them. Hospital medicine is a kind of calling. Like me, each care team vows to serve all lives. Therefore, why don't they explore all the alternatives they can offer to the patients they accept the responsibility to treat? I continue to believe that cutting is not healing. I still cannot fathom the narrow-mindedness of the medical profession.

The Mind Was Never Born. The Mind Has Never Died.

Some doctors showed an interest in my recovery, but not necessarily to discover the therapeutic benefits of my meditations. They listened to me, not without displaying some condescension, and then abruptly listed my case among those unexplained, spontaneous recoveries. While my recovery is all but unexplainable, I still have at my disposal remarks and logical descriptions about what happened that are consistent with a very structured system of thought. In monastic studies, we are trained not only for contemplative meditation but also for dialectics and argumentation. My meditation is not disconnected from a corpus of precise knowledge. Meditation relies on an exhaustive and detailed theoretical basis, one that forms the core of the inner sciences of the subtle body and of the contemplative yoga practices of *tsa-lung*.

I often had the feeling that the doctors at Bellevue Hospital considered my body a series of disconnected spare parts. The doctors were obsessed by the idea of cutting my leg below the knee. This was written in all of their reports and was abbreviated as BKA, for "below knee amputation." In the same way, surgeons will mutilate in the name of saving lives by cutting hands and fingers and removing organs such as the gall bladder, the spleen, or the stomach. But there are other methods of healing. Tibetan medicine, and Chinese or Ayurvedic medicines, use remedies based on plants or natural substances that perfectly restore fractures, treat infected wounds, or reestablish the functions of failing organs.

Since my experience, I have reflected extensively on the system of thought that forms the framework of modern medicine. Of course, modern medicine saves a great number of lives thanks to its mastery of remarkably advanced medical techniques — but its approach was faulty in my case, and probably in other cases, too. The root of the problem, it seems to me, is a total lack of knowledge of the nature of the mind. Medicine's great mistake is to confuse mind and brain.

In the field of health, the medical profession as a whole, from nurses to specialists, considers the existence of the mind to be a function of the brain. Cognitive events are reduced to signals that can be observed thanks to contemporary imaging techniques. Scientists do not consider that the activity of the mind may be different from the brain waves that are printed on their photographs. This is a serious mistake. Even if MRIs or fMRIs actually record the life of the mind, this is only on a rough and very superficial level. We are taught in my tradition that, while the immediate source of physical life comes from the bodies and reproductive systems of our parents, the source of the mind can only be the mind. Physical or organic matter cannot give birth to the mind. An individual's mind arises from mind before the moment of conception; this is an event of consciousness belonging to a stream of consciousness. This has been demonstrated in all Tibetan Buddhist schools. Entire volumes have been written on the nature of the mind, and meditators have realized it through lives dedicated to practice.

When the brain dies, it is called brain death. But does the mind die when the brain dies? This subject has been neglected too often in the West, and it should be the subject of further investigation. All Eastern cultures have examined this question, both in the ancient past and today, and in every field, from popular culture to science to academia. It is crucial that we listen to what they have to say on this subject, which is unanimous:

The mind was never born.
The mind has never died.

Consciousness beyond Sensory Consciousness

I grew up with the examples of yogis who had died, whose hearts had stopped beating, but whose bodies did not begin decaying for another three, sometimes four weeks. During this time, I could see them radiating, giving off fragrances and a warmth at the level of the heart chakra between the lungs. In our tradition, we accept brain death, which corresponds to the very brief moment of death. Breathing stops, but inner winds, and the life of the mind, go on for a period of time. This is estimated to be three days for ordinary people. In the case of yogis who are trained in deep meditations, this life of the mind after death can go on for several weeks.

On a subtle level, the mind is present in the energy body —
the *vajra* body — that we experience thanks to the *tsa-lung* practices. This energy flows inside of, and outside of, the human
body. This energy of universal life is what I used to reconstruct
the blood vessels, the nerves, the cartilage, and the bones of my
ruined ankle. Yet this energy does not come from the brain. This
vital principle of the mind is the creative force that gives life to
our physical cells and our brain cells and keeps them alive. It is
through derivation that the brain, its structure, and its function-
alities are produced. The initial impulse of life, the source of life,
is in the mind.

In yogis, energy continues to inhabit the body as long as they
continue their postmortem meditation. Some of them manage
to match their carnal dimension with the subtle vibration of elements, and they demonstrate *ja-lu* or a "rainbow body." Their
physical body is completely absorbed in a scintillating light with
the colors of the five elements: yellow for the earth, white for
water, red for fire, green for wind, and blue for space.

Other meditators, feeling the moment of their death drawing
near, lock themselves up in a room, while asking not to be disturbed for three weeks. Since the occupation of Tibet, Chinese
soldiers have sometimes forced these doors open and come back
out terror-stricken. They saw, with their own eyes, bodies of old
men that had shrunk to the size of babies. Or they discovered inert
bodies, in a posture of meditation, looking young and lively, even
though the yogis had died hundreds of years earlier. Monks would
have cut their hair, beard, and nails, which would have continued
to grow. Je Tsongkhapa is an example of this; his body was discovered soft and alive in the main chapel of Ganden Monastery.

These processes of transformation or preservation of the
physical body are made possible thanks to the persistence of the
mind's activity in the body. The mind endures after cardiac arrest,

which causes brain death but not the death of the mind. While a corpse decays and becomes pestilent as soon as the flesh is not irrigated, in cases like these, the body remains fresh, the skin is smooth, and it even gives off fragrances. Witnesses often have the impression that the person has become younger, so relaxed is the face. This is only the sign that the person is bathing in the clear light of death, an irradiation of the pure state of the mind when freed from its mental state, or the mental activities that are the origins of suffering.

Following death, the body is in a state of complete rest. There are no more signals of activity in the blood vessels, the gray matter, or the nerves. Therefore, the mind of the yogi gives life to the system of subtle channels, where energies continue to flow in the form of inner winds. The mind is compared to the rider, and the winds to the horse he is riding. Horse and rider, winds and mind, are inseparable.

When a Buddha awakens, his subtle body is present in the very shape of his physical body, completely merged with his energy body. The body of a Buddha is different from that of an ordinary being. It possesses remarkable physical signs that are called the thirty-two major excellent characteristics and the eighty secondary excellent characteristics. The first of these major signs, for example, is that the sole of each foot is adorned with a thousand-spoked wheel, for a being that awakens has always honored and accompanied his master. His palms are adorned in the same way, for he has practiced generosity in a pure and perfect way. Among the minor signs, the hands are as soft as cotton, with clear, deep, and long lines, and they have wide open and clear eyes with thick lashes and well-defined black and white parts, similar to the petals of a lotus flower.

The body of an awakened being is also endowed with miraculous powers, like having "swift feet" that allow him to go somewhere at the speed of thought. Since the mind of a Buddha completely fills his physical body, he only needs to imagine a place for his corporeal energy — of purely spiritual essence — to manifest itself there. An awakened mind is light, the color of gold, with bluish reflections. It is a mind of energy present everywhere and nowhere. It transcends categories of space and time, which are limitations of the mental state. Immeasurable and incandescent, it vibrates in every object, whether animate or inanimate.

This is incomprehensible for Western medicine, a science based on a materialistic approach to healing. It is impossible to detect the activity of the mind — since the level of its manifestation is beyond the most sophisticated techniques of cerebral imagery — so experts in neuroscience conclude too quickly that it's nonexistent, since they believe that what cannot be seen does not exist. The mind is thus confused with the brain, and death is equated with a cessation of brain activity. This is the moment when all crude consciousnesses become ineffective — more precisely, when visual consciousness, auditory consciousness, olfactory consciousness, flavor consciousness, tactile consciousness, and mental consciousness are disconnected from the cognitive decoding processes. The Western scientific world does not acknowledge an autonomous state of consciousness separate from the sensory ones.

Yet, identifying a psychological state isolated and separate from any sensory state makes up the initial practice of *tsa-lung*, which I was trained in from the age of sixteen at Golok Monastery. When I went down to Sera Mey in southern India, I was also taught deep instructions in inner yoga energy. In other words, I had already had roughly twenty years of practice when I embarked upon my healing retreat in New York City. I often meet people who would like to stop medical treatments, hoping to heal on their own through meditation. But they lack the necessary prior training, and I have never encouraged any unprepared person to follow my example.

My education has allowed me to combine the three main levels of Buddhist practice: the religious, or ritualistic level, as a monk; the philosophical level, as a geshe; and the inner sciences level, as a meditator in energy yoga. Such an education involves meditating for tens of thousands of hours, and in my case, I have counted 77,745 hours of pure practice over twenty-five years, without counting the time spent in philosophical studies and debate. This amounts to an average of nine hours a day. Accumulating a significant amount of time practicing is necessary to correct negative habits and replace them with sound attitudes on the three levels of body, speech, and mind. Once inner harmony is found, meditation enables us to become familiar with the more subtle nature of the mind. Such an awakened presence, which we discover in the deepest parts of our thoughts, becomes the object of attention at the root of genuine inner peace, or *shamatha*, which is born from contemplation.

My Recovery Is Not Miraculous

The doctors of Bellevue Hospital have told me that my spontaneous recovery is not unique, which is funny. They were not interested in the improvement of my gangrene, nor did anyone acknowledge having wrongly recommended amputation. However, afterward, some did not hesitate to suggest that I'd experienced a miraculous healing rather than accept that I might have healed thanks to meditation!

This attitude reveals a different unwillingness to understand. I am a Buddhist monk, but I do not claim that Buddhist practice is the only path toward healing. We each develop the potential of our mind in a specific way, by following the spiritual path that corresponds to the development of our own karma. Is it not said in the scriptures that there are eighty-four thousand doors to enter the doctrine of liberation?

For me, there is no doubt that other religions, and other meditative practices — like Reiki or qigong, for example — can heal illnesses as serious as cancer or AIDS. As a matter of fact, it is not one or another tradition that brings healing, it is in knowing how to use the energy of our mind. Whatever method, whatever religion, whether we are Christian, Muslim, or Hindu, each system has developed a therapeutic approach. Mine is suitable for me; it includes meditations on light and emptiness in a transformative dimension, or *bodhicitta*, the spirit of altruistic Awakening. But I know that this approach, which has saved me, is far from unique. It makes me happy that human beings have different conceptions, since it is good to be able to choose and enjoy the method most appropriate and most efficient for ourselves. Ignoring the nature of the mind, which they confuse with brain activity, doctors have sometimes asked me to bring them proof that I recovered thanks to meditation. There is no lack of proofs, but the proofs are not coherent with their reference system or interpretive grid. They don't fit their worldview.

For a long time, scientists believed that neurons were determined and unchanged from birth, but they have recently accepted the notion of brain plasticity. This is important progress. However, according to the inner sciences of *tsa-lung*, the mind is infinitely more flexible and mobile than the brain. Because of its lightness and fluidity, the mind can be compared to a bubble of water. A water bubble does not cease fluctuating, just like the mind. If the mind is trained, it becomes possible to transform it. That is why it is important to cultivate, and to maintain, positive emotions such as love, benevolence, open-mindedness, and the wisdom that arises in contact with truth.

Before dying and entering the in-between state, or *bardo*, the rough elements of sensory consciousnesses are eliminated. We are then given a chance, in that ultimate moment of human life, to be revealed the true nature of the mind. It appears in full light, not in its veiled state, when brain death occurs. It is important to know that will happen and, during our lifetime, to learn how to use our mind advisedly. If we continuously allow ourselves to be absorbed in material objects, without controlling our wishes, our attachments, or our anger, the states of mind causing veils will linger beyond physical life, after death. Once our mind has left its corporeal support, it will become extremely difficult to transform such mental afflictions and to eradicate fear, anger, or jealousy from our stream of consciousness.

On the other hand, if in this life we practice energy yoga, and we merge our mind with the mind of a pure and perfect master, this praiseworthy state of mind will automatically appear at the moment of death. Or if, during this life, we have bathed our consciousness in the contemplation of sacred art, whether it is paintings or statues of awakened beings, while reciting prayers and mantras, such positive dispositions will be with us after death. And if we manage to recognize our mind, we will be instantly freed from the cycle of rebirth in conditioned lives.

Someday, in this life, I hope to do in-depth teaching on the reality of the mind, as my experience has revealed it to me. If I can convince doctors of the importance of the mind in the process of physical recovery, they will be able to heal in a better way a greater number of people. The complementary nature of contemporary medical techniques and of spiritual traditions and the ancestral wisdom of the inner sciences seems to me a good way, full of promise. It will enable people to blossom, for it allows people to integrate the essential dimension of the life of the mind with the art of medical treatment.

Menla Thödöl Ling, the "Medicine Buddha Garden"

After my recovery, I did not cease offering my merits and prayers to found a center in the West dedicated to the promotion of the inner sciences of peace and healing. I did not know how quickly these wishes would come true, but ever since my dream at the age of thirteen, in which I followed Maitreya Buddha and said yes to Je Tsongkhapa, I have vowed to fundamentally serve beings — all beings.

I have offered my life to relieve all beings from various forms of suffering, be it physical or mental distress. I have always firmly believed in the achievement of this goal, and my intentions were only reinforced by my experience with illness and suffering. Armed with this conviction, I have not ceased practicing, day after day; my only goal is to transmit the methods that have allowed me to heal.

But it takes all conditions to be combined. I understood they were on the day I met Sofia Stril-Rever. Our meeting was the result of the ripening of a karma going back several lives ago. In the past, many journalists, writers, and film directors tried to convince me to write my story. But I was not sure they would grasp it in all of its depth. My soul links with Sofia are such that I chose to entrust my story to her. I entrusted to her the launching of my teaching program "Experiencing Peace and Inner Healing,"* since I know she is motivated by genuine compassion. She herself has worked to elucidate deep levels of teachings on mind and energy. At Kirti Monastery in Dharamsala, a great *vajra* master taught her the Kalachakra Tantra system, a supreme and basic teaching of Tibetan medicine. With the master's guidance, and the Dalai

---

* A three-year program teaching *shamatha*, "Experiencing Peace and Inner healing," started in March 2015 with the first followers, and many others have since joined the program.

Lama's blessing, Sofia translated from Sanskrit, for the first time in a Western language, the book of the subtle body in the Kalachakra Tantra. She has also recorded the spiritual autobiography of the Dalai Lama, titled *My Spiritual Journey*, as well as his book *My Appeal to the World*, both of which recount his fight for justice, truth, and peace. Sofia has often sung the Heart Sutra in Sanskrit at the opening of teaching sessions of the Dalai Lama, and she has adapted the melodies of Tibetan prayers to their French translation. When I heard her for the first time, I was moved to recognize the vibration of these songs in a Western language.

At the end of May 2013, she invited me for my first teachings in Europe at an enchanted place in the branches of the Eure River that is inhabited by wild swans. One of them — whom Sofia named Asanga, or "Without Attachment" — came near her when she called him and nibbled in her hand. Migratory birds often stop on the banks of the willow-bordered pond. I had hardly gone through the entrance gate when I heard the warbling of a cuckoo, a bird of my childhood that remains dear to my heart. I had not heard it in exactly twenty-three years, since I had left my country. The call of the cuckoo was a sign. It told me that the soul of Tibet is alive in the area.

Today, I continue to develop my curriculum on inner sciences and contemplative healing yoga practices here, and I originally suggested to Sofia to call the place Menla Thödöl Ling, the "Garden of Liberation through Listening to the Medicine Buddha," or more simply the "Medicine Buddha Garden." I really believe that a sincerely motivated practitioner can experience pure land on these premises and take his or her first steps toward liberation of suffering.

BOOK TWO

MAY EVERYONE HEAR
WHAT THEY NEED TO AWAKEN

By Sofia Stril-Rever

Who looks outside, dreams.
Who looks inside, awakes.

— CARL GUSTAV JUNG

CHAPTER ONE

The Sutra of the Heroic March

How Can One Write the Story of Someone Who Has No Ego Left?

"Sofia, I cannot answer all your questions!"

Rinpoche bursts out laughing. His joyful energy is infectious, and I laugh with him. He blushes, buries his head in his hands, or hides behind his garnet-colored shawl. Then he shows himself again, energetically rubbing his shaved head. A moment of silence follows. He bends his head forward and looks up at me. We stop talking. He speaks to me first without speaking. After a certain time, at last, in his yogi eyes, eyes with a contemplative radiance offered entirely without desire to grasp or gain power over the world, I can read a gleam of assent. Rinpoche starts speaking slowly, in a deep voice, in rough English. He articulates words that, though lacking basic syntax, are filled with unexpected depth.

It is a remarkable speech. For Phakyab Rinpoche is a *muni*, as was the "Sage of the Shakya,"* and along with him, all the masters

---

* This phrase is the direct translation of "Shakyamuni Buddha," or the historic Buddha. The term *muni* can mean, variously, sage, saint, holy person, seer, ascetic, monk, hermit, or recluse, and the name *Shakyamuni* literally means "sage of the Shakya tribe."

of the beginning of Buddhism. In schools in ancient times, it was claimed that Buddha would not discourse to teach, but would only utter a single sound, a sound in which everyone would hear what they needed to awake.

Phakyab Rinpoche is also a master, trained in philosophical debate, dialectics, and argumentation. Therefore, as he speaks, he goes from articulating very supported ideas — such as when reasoning on the nature of mind — to disclosing, in bits and pieces, and with a sense of modesty, his own story and journey toward Awakening.

"It, it, it…it is tiring to speak about oneself! And about oneself again!"

Rinpoche sighs. This is obviously the very first time he has endeavored to tell the story of his life. He is disconcerted, and at times disconcerting. At the beginning, I wonder if we will be able to collect his memories. How can one write the biography of someone who has no ego left?

Between what is said and not said, I gather scattered bits. We reconstruct the puzzle of the beginning of his life as an exile. In February 2014, I join him in New York City, and together we go back in time during the icy winter of the East Coast. At Bellevue Hospital, we meet the manager of the Program for Survivors of Torture, where Tibetans, Chinese, Iranians, Serbs, Congolese, Sudanese, Cameroonians, etc., rub shoulders. I hear all languages spoken in these halls, where the care team helps survivors of barbarity reconstruct. There are no borders on the map of people who have been denied humanity. Rinpoche discovered the world, with his brothers and sisters in suffering, in this very special health care service of a New York City hospital.

We go together to Pema Dorje's former apartment, at 265 Manhattan Avenue, near the Williamsburg Bridge. Rinpoche has not been back since his recovery. Is it a coincidence? Mr. Lee, the Chinese landlord, comes back home precisely when we arrive, and he opens the door for us. Rinpoche introduces himself, but Mr. Lee, with a blank look, does not seem to remember him — or maybe he does not want to remember, since he is disturbed by my camera and my recorder.

At Tibet House, we meet Robert Thurman, who is my publisher and friend in the United States. Robert is very forthcoming about Rinpoche, for he had played a very special part as a messenger to the Dalai Lama. Later on, I speak with Marina Illich on Skype, since she now lives in California, and little by little, I put faces to the names that Rinpoche mentions. The story of his healing comes alive.

Meeting with Dr. Zoran Josipovic

I am expecting a lot from our meeting with Dr. Zoran Josipovic.[*] A researcher in neurosciences at New York University, he is also the founding director of the Nonduality Institute. His mission is to offer meditation programs on the subtle nature of consciousness, that "vast, unchanging, ineffable expanse, equal to space, timeless and innately present in all sentient beings," to quote the great Tibetan yogi Longchenpa.[†]

We meet in a bar near his laboratory. In the subdued lights, I almost can't make out Dr. Josipovic's prominent features, but I can see the intensity of his eyes. They alight with passion for his research in contemplative neurosciences and with joy at seeing

---

[*] At New York University, Dr. Zoran Josipovic studies the effects of contemplative practices on the organization of the brain in order to better understand the nature of consciousness and the self. At the Nonduality Institute (www.nondualityinstitute .org), he directs a contemplative science laboratory and teaches meditation.

[†] Longchen Rabjampa Drimé Öser, also known as Longchenpa, lived in the fourteenth century. This great master of the Nyingma School of Buddhism, called the "Omniscient," was revered as an emanation of Manjushri, the Bodhisattva of Wisdom.

Phakyab Rinpoche again, to whom he speaks with marked defer-
ence. His face brightens as he confides to me: "I have been practicing meditation for some thirty years now, mostly in the Tibetan
Buddhist tradition. I have met many masters, but none has introduced me to meditation in a way as inspiring and refreshing as Rinpoche. He speaks about his healing with astounding simplicity!"

Dr. Josipovic has heard about healings that have been called
"miraculous," and he has directly witnessed unexplainable supernatural phenomena. However, he claims he has never met someone
as willing as Rinpoche to talk openly about an event as extraordinary as his healing, explaining precisely and in detail how it occurred. This is why Dr. Josipovic asked Rinpoche to participate
in research that his team is carrying out with experienced meditators at New York University's Cognitive Neurophysiology Laboratory.

Phakyab Rinpoche jokes about the very inappropriate conditions for meditation in the sarcophagus-like fMRI machine. Nevertheless, in the experiment, he did his best to meditate inside it.
He says lying down was an unfamiliar position, and the noises
of this powerful machine photographing his brain were very
unpleasant. But he endured these constraints willingly, for the
Dalai Lama unceasingly encourages Tibetan lamas to contribute
to research that explores neurology and meditation — especially
lamas who, like Rinpoche, have accumulated an impressive number of hours of practice.

"Some yogis," Dr. Josipovic admits, "have at times had the
feeling of having their head stuck in the drum of a washing machine set to spin dry at a thousand revolutions per minute! It is
true that such an environment is ill-adapted to contemplative
meditation, and it could be detrimental to the experiment. But in
Rinpoche's case, we were surprised to see that he very quickly

became absorbed in advanced states of meditation, showing an uncommon capacity to bring about total peace in his mind."

For Dr. Josipovic, studying meditation through cerebral imaging is a major advance. It has allowed the emergence of a new field, that of contemplative neurosciences, and it has very quickly yielded promising results. Indeed, their research has already revealed, on the one hand, great clinical potential and, on the other hand, an ability to answer questions about the nature of mental phenomena, such as neuroplasticity and epigenetic changes in the brain.

The therapeutic effects of full consciousness and compassion meditation do not need to be proven anymore. Instead, the goal of Dr. Josipovic's original and innovative research is to identify the cerebral alterations that result from nondual meditation, or clear light meditation, in Tibetan Buddhism. This very subtle state of consciousness is described as a thought before thinking, a latent awakened presence, underlying every cognitive event and every mental process.

"Such a level of consciousness is not yet known in Western science," remarks Dr. Josipovic. "What studies in cerebral imaging show us concerns the neuronal correlates of consciousness, or the changes of activity and organization of the brain according to different types of meditative contemplation. Studies can't yet explain, once and for all, the ontological status of clear light, for example, but for each state of consciousness, there is a corresponding neuronal correlate, or a minimal set of specific neuronal events. Starting from this premise, and from the more recent discoveries on brain functioning, we have worked out a theoretical framework and identified a network of cerebral areas in the precuneus, situated in the superior parietal lobe. This area seems to form the neuronal correlate of clear light. Other research is being considered in order to grasp more complex changes associated with nondual aspects of meditation, when they become widespread throughout the brain, thereby showing their integration in the cerebral network."

Has clear consciousness made its way from the secrecy of Himalayan caves to the high-tech labs of New York City?

"This kind of study is an everyday challenge to take up," Dr. Josipovic observes regretfully. "The scientific establishment accuses us of using science to enhance primitive religious beliefs. As for meditators, they sometimes blame us for using them, and their traditions, to further our research, without respecting the deep meaning of their spiritual practices. To me, I think the greatest challenge is that the mapping of consciousness — which people have explored over several centuries of meditative experience and philosophical debate in different schools, Hindu as well as Buddhist — cannot easily be translated into the nomenclature of Western cognitive sciences."

Dr. Josipovic speaks with the firm belief of one who has seen and who knows. His research in cerebral imaging has made him a well-informed witness of what yogis train all their lives to contemplate at the time of their death: the clear light of bliss that illuminates the passage into in-between lives. When body and mind separate, it is indeed as if a veil were torn open. The primordial purity of wisdom is not hidden anymore by sensory perceptions and mental productions. It reflects the radiating brilliance of its compassionate energy. Entire volumes of Buddhist tantras, and their commentaries, have described that very subtly, or they have sung it like Padmasambhava in this verse on the marvels of natural clear light:

> Clear light, that has its source within itself, and that was
> never born since origins, is child of clear light, itself
> without parent — oh wonder!

This wisdom, that has its source within itself, was
    created by no one — oh wonder!
It was never born, and nothing can cause its death — oh
    wonder!
Though it is perfectly visible, it cannot be seen — oh
    wonder!
Though it has wandered in the samsara, nothing wrong
    happened to it — oh wonder!
Though it is within each of us, nobody has acknowledged
    it — oh wonder!
And you still continue to hope elsewhere for some other
    fruit — oh wonder!
Though it is most essentially yours, you seek for it
    elsewhere — oh wonder!

Twenty-First-Century Monk

After returning from New York City, I allow the impressions of the past — one that does not belong to me, but that my mind reviews so that it can be translated into words — to settle. I recall the skyline and the cityscapes of Manhattan, Brooklyn, and Queens, which I explored with Rinpoche by my side; the corridors of Bellevue Hospital, which we paced up and down together; and the meetings with people, unknown to me, who cared and supported Rinpoche in the trying times of his beginnings in New York City, then in the stages of his recovery, and then in his first teachings in the United States. I allow myself to tread the paths of his life. They take me far from myself, into unexplored regions — yet they bring me closer to myself. In them, I discover teachings of magnified humanity and extremes of sublimated thought, for they are freed from mental veils.

    I let myself be swept away in the invisible dimensions inhabited by Phakyab Rinpoche, and I come back to reality through the channel of sensitive memories, endlessly going over images, words, gazes, and silences. Moments I've lived start resonating with Rinpoche's mind. His story takes shape in my story. It comes together in the trajectory from the Himalayan peaks to the Manhattan skyscrapers, fluctuating between an immemorial anchorage in the ages of the Earth and the futuristic creations of a vulnerable — because it is uprooted — West.

As the contours of Phakyab Rinpoche's life become more precise, my questions become more targeted. As we talk, I am the direct witness to the downfall of years of silence and self-censorship. One day, Rinpoche acknowledges: "The Dalai Lama says times have changed. Twenty-first-century monks have to explain that they encounter spiritual achievements. Otherwise, nobody will listen to them. We used to show tremendous respect for the most unpretentious people. We used to consider that, when everything is understood, there is nothing more to say. A wise man would remain silent. Nowadays, it is exactly the opposite."

But I have another request. I also want to hear the story of his childhood, for I sense that the first years of his life hold the keys to essential understanding. At first, Rinpoche seems dumbfounded. Why am I so interested in that period? He intends to start his story at the age of thirty-seven, with his arrival in New York City and the start of his illness. I am trespassing the boundaries of an intimate and secret territory.

I explain to Rinpoche that the Dalai Lama has told me about his upbringing. Without any hesitation, comfortable with himself and laughing heartily, the Dalai Lama explained how he would squabble with his older brother in the palanquin that took them from eastern Tibet to Lhasa. He always made sure his brother would be punished, when the rough and uncoordinated movements of the children threatened to destabilize the porters. He also revealed to me that he would eat hard-boiled eggs at his mother's in the Norbulingka residence, and that he would often leave the Potala in the morning, firmly resolved not to go back at dusk. The Dalai Lama shared other, similar episodes, taken from the liveliness of his memories, and I also want Rinpoche to tell me what kind of child he had been. I want to follow him as a teenager, and as a young monk, to elucidate the process that paved the way for his healing. It is impossible to write the story of a disembodied being and pretend his life started at almost forty.

Rinpoche considers it. The example of the Dalai Lama helps him overcome his reserve. Undoubtedly, his fits of giggles over his memories help him lift his restrictions and transform his initial disinterest at narrating his life — until he eventually opens up. Then he recounts anecdotes one after the other, without my asking for them. They form the network of a tale that he has never before shared, not even with his relatives or close friends. I am tremendously grateful to him for his trust, and we agree that nothing will be published without his agreement. Once it's finished, we reread the whole manuscript word for word.

The Tibet of Amputated Children.
The Tibet of Human Torches.

The first time I heard about Phakyab Rinpoche was in Washington, DC. I had been invited by Robert Thurman to give a lecture and translate the teachings of the Dalai Lama, who was giving the great initiation of Kalachakra. I arrived very early every morning, and by 6 AM, I was meditating to the sound of the entrancing ritual, which continued for two weeks in the presence of the Dalai Lama. There were few people at the crack of dawn, and seated in the first row, my neighbor was a pretty young woman with a moving face.

Sonia Tita Puopolo told me her remarkable story. She is the daughter of one of the victims of the first plane that crashed into the World Trade Center on September 11, 2001. A ring with several rows of diamonds glittered on her finger. This engagement ring was found intact, two years after the dramatic event, on her mother's finger, under the tons of rubble of Ground Zero. This improbable discovery — which she considered a miraculous sign of maternal love from beyond — helped Sonia transcend the pain of bereavement. This experience overcoming suffering inspired her to write a book, *Sonia's Ring: 11 Ways to Heal Your Heart*, which acknowledges that we all, in our lives, go through 9/11 situations. Citing the world's various wisdom traditions, the book answers the questions: How can we face a situation when everything is collapsing? How can we find reasons for hope? How can we transform suffering?

In Washington, DC, Sonia told me about Phakyab Rinpoche. His story is part of the current tragedy of Tibet, where amputations are a political reality. The first time I went to the Tibetan Children's Villages in Dharamsala, the Dalai Lama's sister, Jetsun Pema, introduced me to Dorje Tseten. This shy teenager, whose face intermittently brightened with joy, stopped being a child at the age of five. That was when his mother entrusted her son to smugglers, so he could join the exiled Tibetan community in India that had developed around His Holiness the Dalai Lama. She hoped he would have the life of a monk, which frees one from the worst karmas. For the modest sum of two thousand yuan (less than three hundred American dollars), the smugglers were supposed to take the boy to a relative in Kathmandu. They would follow the narrow path that goes through the Himalayan barrier down to the "Gorges of Hell," toward Zhangmu, the border town where Tibetan, Chinese, Nepalese, and Indian merchants bump into tourists from all over the world.

But the smugglers abandoned Dorje Tseten by night in the vicinity of the Nyalam Tong La pass, which is at an elevation of almost 17,000 feet. When he woke up, he was lying on a flat stone, alone, absolutely alone. He was like a little snow prince, frozen stiff under his *chupa* lined with sheepskin, a multicolored scarf around his neck. He spent two days there, with no water and no food, his body becoming stiffer in the shroud of icy wind. Then a humming pierced the sky, and the little boy got up and waved his scarf at this providential helicopter. The passengers saw him, and the aircraft landed nearby. Dorje Tseten was saved.

The tourist couple who rescued him took him for medical treatment to the American hospital in Kathmandu. His feet had frozen, and all of his toes had to be amputated. He learned how to walk again by using little leather orthopedic shoes that were placed inside his tennis shoes and supported his feet. Dorje Tseten was lucky compared to other Tibetan children. In the Himalayan snowfields, some lose a leg or a hand when they do not lose their life.

Though only thirteen when we met, he displayed a heroic resistance, saying to me with conviction: "It is better to be in India, near the Dalai Lama, without toes, than being in Lhasa with all of my toes!"

The Tibet of amputated children.

The Tibet of human torches.

On the Roof of the World, women and men, young and in the prime of life, monks and laymen, make the supreme sacrifice of their life. They immolate themselves, choosing the torture of a slow and painful death to protest and say no to the all-mighty Chinese dictatorship, which the world silently allows. On September 26, 2011, at the age of eighteen, Lobsang Kunchok, a monk from Kirti Monastery, set himself ablaze in Ngaba in eastern Tibet. The People's Armed Police extinguished the fire and took his still-living, charred body away. Six months later, in March 2012, sources of information in exile broadcast the news that Lobsang Kunchok had had both legs and both arms amputated. He was in detention in a military hospital, and yet, despite his condition, he was still being subjected to physical abuse, blows, and ill treatment. Several members of his family were also imprisoned and tortured; they were accused of complicity in his immolation, which is considered a "crime against state security."

When I heard the story of Phakyab Rinpoche, whose gangrene occurred after the brutality of an arbitrary arrest, it symbolized for me the sufferings of the Tibetan people, who have been deprived of their fundamental liberties for sixty years, and the resignation of the great Western democracies, which have not assumed their duty to defend universal human rights. But Rinpoche's recovery also includes the mystical dimension of sutras.

The Sutra of the Heroic March

In many instances in his former lives, the Buddha happened to cut off one of his limbs or a part of his body as an offering to starving beings, since generosity is the first of the perfections of the path toward Awakening. In an unconditional form, it can go as far as amputation, the ultimate sacrifice that sanctifies the soul when it is offered for the well-being of all beings.

For instance, in one of his lives, the Buddha was Princess Rupavati. One day, she severed her breasts to feed a malnourished woman who was about to eat her newborn baby. Or in another life, the Blessed was embodied as the son of a merchant, Chandraprabha. Driven by extreme compassion, he went to a mass grave and gave his body away to feed hungry ghosts. In the shape of birds of prey, they first pecked away at his eyes, and then they dismembered him and devoured him completely. The Buddha was also the young Brahmin Brahmaprabha, who bled his arm to revive a starving tigress. When she had recovered enough strength, he gave her his body so she could feed her five little children. Such amputations are initiatory steps toward perfect Awakening, and after each one of his mutilations, the Buddha recovered his physical integrity.

The Sutra of the Heroic March is another example, and Phakyab Rinpoche's story called it to mind immediately. This passage of the scriptures describes how, before Awakening, the Buddha was the ascetic Kshantivadin, the "Follower of Patience." One day, the king of Kalinga, along with his court, went on a hunting expedition not far from the ascetic's place of meditation in the forest, which had the same name. When his queens caught sight of Kshantivadin, they were enthralled by the peace radiating from him. The king — who had continued on in pursuit of the game — later found them at his feet, drinking in his words. Overcome by uncontrolled jealousy, the king accused the renouncer of wanting to seduce them. Trying to spark the anger of the Follower of Patience, the king cut his ears, then his nose, and then each of his limbs in succession. Finally, the wise man of the forest answered the provocation of the king, saying: "If I have completely eliminated anger within me, may my arms and legs testify to it by immediately growing back! May my body become whole again! But if I am lying, and still have anger within me, may my hands and feet not reunite with my body! May my nose and ears not grow back!"

With these words, his body reconstructed completely. After witnessing this phenomenon, the king accused Kshantivadin of being a demon, and he brandished his saber to cut his head off. But at that very moment, the guardians made a hailstorm shower on him, and he was annihilated. The future Buddha then prayed for the monarch to be saved. Kshantivadin forgave the king and promised to lead him to Awakening, as soon as he himself reached perfect enlightenment. This vow became true. For the day Prince

Siddhartha became the Awakened Shakyamuni, the first person he delivered from suffering was his torturer from the forest, the king of Kalinga.

Before I personally met Phakyab Rinpoche, just from the stories I heard about him, I found myself thinking of the unconditional generosity the Buddha displayed in his former lives. How could one not make the connection? I felt moved by this lama's strength of mind, which allowed him to flee from Chinese prisons and to walk across the Himalayas with a wounded ankle. I was moved by the strength of his compassion, which gave him the power to reconstruct his gangrened leg. And I was moved by his magnanimity toward those who tortured him by forgiving them and praying for them. Reaching that stage implies a spirit of unconditional love combined with a deep fulfillment of voidness, or emptiness. If Phakyab Rinpoche had not transcended attachment to his physical body, how could he have avoided amputation or death, the unavoidable consequences of gangrene?

His meditation was successful because he perfectly experienced the link of interdependence that unites all living beings. If one fails to integrate this within the wisdom of experience, then illusion and self-attachment do not allow universal energy to be channeled and combined with inner winds. Yet only through such a process was Rinpoche able to rebuild his cartilages, his bones, and the tissues of his gangrened right foot. Today, Rinpoche feels with absolutely certainty that his healing represents only the achievement of a relative goal. The ultimate goal is Awakening.

Padampa Sangye's Mantra

There was more still. As I discovered the remarkable story of Phakyab Rinpoche, his recovery echoed an experience of disabling neurological illness that affected me for seven years. It started in 1998, and the doctors I consulted were unable to make a diagnosis. My symptoms were those of a brain tumor, but the MRI proved negative.

"You have a beautiful cortex!" the radiologist commented as she scrutinized my cerebral X-rays, a magnifying glass in her hand. I was relieved, but since the examination revealed nothing, it was impossible to name the reason for my symptoms, and I was offered no treatment. After not detecting any physical causes, the doctors advised that I seek psychiatric treatment, which I refused. I was prescribed powerful neuroleptics that made me fall asleep in broad daylight. I very quickly stopped taking them and tried homeopathic treatments and acupuncture without success. I repeatedly made all kinds of medical appointments.

That is, until I accepted this health issue and the everyday problems it caused me. Oddly, I did not think this illness would wear me out, which would have been logical. On the contrary, I was convinced that the illness would wear itself out, and that when the time came, I would meet the therapist who would help me recover my health. Armed with this conviction, I learned how to live with these disabling symptoms, while I carried on translating the Kalachakra Tantra from Sanskrit into French. Through this work, in combination with teachings I received at Kirti Monastery in Dharamsala, I was revealed the depth of tantric meditation, and the experience of my illness became anchored in spiritual practice.

One day in 2003, I saw the picture of a lama doctor and yogi, Dr. Nida Chenagtsang.* I instinctively felt he could cure me. He was teaching traditional Tibetan medicine, namely *ku-nye*, a massage that stimulates the energetic body. Two years later, in the fall of 2005, I enrolled in one of his seminars on mantra therapy, and afterward I asked him for a massage session.

---

* A graduate from the medical school in Lhasa, Dr. Nida Chenagtsang founded in 2006 the International Academy for Traditional Tibetan Medicine (www.iattm.net).

Dr. Nida took my pulse, following the traditional Tibetan medical protocol, and concluded that no massage would help me. On the other hand, he suggested I chant a certain mantra, which he transmitted to me, explaining the conditions for practicing it. Puzzled, and somewhat disappointed, I nevertheless strictly followed his recommendations. In the pitch dark night of the new moon in November 2005, I chanted a sixteen-syllable mantra six thousand times. In the dark, while chanting, I made the break sounds click, to cut off mental conditioning and establish the mind in its loving and dazzling basis.

During the following weeks, the symptoms did not reappear. They never came back. I was cured. Anxious to go deeper into the subject, I studied mantra therapy, a medical version of mantra yoga, and translated into French Dr. Nida's teachings. After several years of practice, he allowed me to transmit the healing mantras that form the basis of mantra therapy. In Tibet, these mantras never replace medical treatments, but they are considered treasures in the heart of awakened beings, and they give support when someone is sick or at the end of life, with remarkable results. If the right conditions are satisfied, they can heal the physical body, as was the case for me, but the aim is ultimate healing.

When I finally met Phakyab Rinpoche in May 2013, he asked me about the mantra that healed me. I answered that I continued to chant it regularly at night during a new moon, and that it belongs to the healing transmissions of the great Mahasiddha, Padampa Sangye. I have a portrait of him with his hair in a bun like a yogi, wearing a bone necklace. He is hitting a tantric drum and blowing into a flute made from a human femur, inviting demons, harmful spirits, and lost souls to come feed on the nectar of wisdom.

Phakyab Rinpoche smiled and remained silent. I asked him if he knew Padampa Sangye and if he was familiar with this mantra.

He smiled again and still said nothing. A year later, Rinpoche told me that he was recognized as one of the emanations of that accomplished yogi. What an unfathomable power of karma! The fruit, born of causes and conditions we are not aware of, is secretly formed in the depths of time incarnate. When it matures, no obstacle can ever oppose its manifestation.

By matching up dates, I noticed that our paths had already crossed in this life several times. The first time was in 2003, in Bodhgaya, during one of the Dalai Lama's teachings. It happened again in 2008 in Dharamsala, in 2010 in southern India, and at last in Washington, DC, in 2011. We had been in the same places, at the same dates, near Kundun. We had probably seen each other, but without meeting. As I expressed surprise, Rinpoche only answered: "The causes and conditions were not gathered. We have met many times, in many lives. The time has come now. There are important things we have to do together in this incarnation."

Eight years earlier, Padampa Sangye had entered my life and physically cured me thanks to his mantra. Now Padampa Sangye was back as Phakyab Rinpoche, and during his first teachings centered on ultimate healing, he made a promise: "The Buddha is not to be sought far or outside of you. Awakened nature is within you. You don't know yet how to look inside of yourself because you are too attached to appearance, which is manifested outside of yourself. Awakening is within the reach of your breaths." My voice faltered. I had a hard time finishing the translation. I had already heard such words from other masters. But borne from his experience of Awakening, Rinpoche's teaching struck another chord. I understood that he could lead me to the hidden heart of the spiritual path.

Every meditative practice, under the covering of words and visualizations, conceals deep mysteries, the basic principle of which remains hidden. No word can reveal it. Until the day when the mental state is pacified at last, and it is delivered in a state of consciousness unified with primal wisdom whose master embodies experience. Then is disclosed the nature of the mind's secrecy, the ultimate guru. No mystery anymore. Everything is revealed.

As this intuition arose, and though we hardly knew each other, I accepted Phakyab Rinpoche's request: "Sofia, you wrote the Dalai Lama's *Spiritual Autobiography* and his *Appeal to the World*? Maybe you could write the story of my healing? I will be completely healed only once this book is written."

CHAPTER TWO

An Exceptionally Powerful Healing

The Medical Point of View of Dr. Lionel Coudron

"Abandoned, Phakyab Rinpoche felt abandoned by the doctors of Bellevue Hospital."

Such is Dr. Lionel Coudron's immediate comment when he starts reading the first few pages of Phakyab Rinpoche's medical file. To assess the case of his atypical recovery, Rinpoche thought it would be a good idea to go see Dr. Coudron, who attended Rinpoche's first lecture in Paris and whom we had the pleasure of meeting afterward.

My eyes meet Dr. Coudron's very blue and deeply therapeutic eyes. We are in his office on Avenue d'Iéna in Paris in the headquarters of the Yoga Therapy Institute, which he founded in 1993. To reach his office, one has to go through a rotunda with mirrored walls. When crossing this space, it is impossible not to think that one comes here to have one's true self revealed. The mirror, just like the mind calmed by meditation, reflects all the appearances of the world without grasping any.

"I welcome patients with serious illnesses for whom hospital medicine offers demanding medical protocols. They would like to heal thanks to yoga. I remain a doctor, as well as being a yoga teacher, and I warn them: Others have come to see me with the same request. Unfortunately, they are not here anymore to talk about it."

Dr. Coudron offers an accompanying program and feels it is his duty not to give up on his patients. He believes it's the patient's responsibility whether or not to follow chemotherapy or radiation therapy, and he warns them about the risks if they cease their treatment — all while making the very precious promise to be by their side and go through the hardship of illness with them. I tell myself that, to have met such a doctor, his patients have an excellent karma. Dr. Coudron knows how to tune in to an energetic and spiritual dimension that helps the person mobilize all their healing potential.

"When I heard about Phakyab Rinpoche's first lecture in Paris, 'Healing through Meditation,' I immediately felt intrigued," remembers Dr. Coudron.

Seated at the far end of the room, Dr. Coudron was increasingly captivated by Rinpoche's words. He said, "I was deeply moved by his story. Rinpoche was telling some hundred people about his unique, incredible experience. He was smiling and full of attention. I could feel, deep inside me, that he was supplying us with an exceptional testimony and, in a disconcertingly natural way, as simply as possible!"

Dr. Coudron does not hesitate to call Phakyab Rinpoche's recovery a "miracle." He has never been confronted with "such a powerful phenomenon," he says. "Even though I have twice had the privilege of recording unexplained recoveries from cancer — which taught me that anything can happen — I had never seen a pathology, whose normal evolution should be lethal, evolve this way. I had, unfortunately, been more often the witness of catastrophes when some yoga teachers whom I knew had rejected conventional medicine. Though I know, from having studied miracles and the placebo effect, that the body is endowed with everything it needs to cure and self-cure, Rinpoche's testimony did not leave me indifferent."

I am surprised to hear a doctor using the word *miracle* when, for Rinpoche, his healing falls within the province of rigorous logic, even if it involves subtle energies. The channels Rinpoche visualizes, and the winds that he masters, are recorded on anatomical charts of the yogic body that are as precise as anatomical charts of the physical body. His healing process was not sudden, and it cannot be compared with instantaneous miracles in Lourdes or in Fatima. For three years, Rinpoche practiced systematic meditation to reconstruct his gangrenous leg and his crumbled spine. I suggest understanding the word *miracle* in its etymological meaning as "something that deserves to be looked at." I say to Dr. Coudron, "A miracle is the mirror of the invisible. As a reflection of the unthinkable, a miracle reflects the ineffable. Doesn't a miracle make us look beyond words? Think beyond thought?"

Dr. Coudron agrees, replying: "When I say *miracle*, I really mean an astonishing and unpredictable event — not a miracle in the Christian sense of the word, resulting from external intervention. This is why I like talking about little everyday miracles. Life is the greatest miracle, the universe, its birth, consciousness, the sun rising, the rain falling, are all miracles linked with a succession of events that are each time incredible. A human being is a miracle. And all this commands enthusiasm and wonder. It is in this sense that Rinpoche's healing is a miracle. A miracle of life, and of its possibilities, that forces us once more to marvel."

I have spoken to other doctors about Phakyab Rinpoche's recovery who have been surprised that it took him three years to heal. Undoubtedly, they were surprised because they could not file his healing into the category of spontaneous miracles that are recorded by various religions in the world.

"Why did it not happen immediately?" they ask skeptically.

Dr. Coudron suggests reformulating this question: "Why immediately and not three years? How could it have been any better? Would it have convinced one more person to practice meditation?"

He continues: "Personally, I do not believe it at all. On the contrary, if his healing had been immediate, it would have been in the realm of the *impossible*. Whereas in the case of Phakyab Rinpoche, what happened involves us all the more as it is the result of assiduous practice, and not of intense and punctual faith. He shows us a path that is in the realm of what is *possible* through training. If I say I have never played soccer, and that the first time I do, I kick a goal against the best team in the world, nobody will believe they have the slightest chance of achieving that. It is obvious that it will not reoccur. If, on the contrary, I explain that I started soccer and have trained for many years to become the best striker in the world, everyone will acknowledge that it is also possible for others. Even if everyone knows that they cannot become the best striker against the best team in the world, everyone knows they can train to their own level and enjoy playing and kicking goals.

"It is the same for Phakyab Rinpoche. In Rinpoche's healing, what is important is not so much the goal but the path he took to reach it. This path consists in developing compassion and a capacity for concentration applied with benevolence to our body. It could not have occurred as if by magic nor in an instant. Phakyab Rinpoche shows us the path of a practice. If we implement it, results will be achieved. Not by chance, but through training. If I want to climb Mount Everest, I need a good amount of training. If I want to hike a few days in the mountain, a less-sophisticated training may be enough. Phakyab Rinpoche shows us that what he did is accessible to anyone in their own life. If I meditate — if only a little bit — I will see its benefits. But for that, I need to sit down, understand my condition, and decide to change it."

Healing through Compassion

To interpret an event that modern science cannot explain and that reason can't account for, Dr. Coudron suggests hypotheses that upset classic dogmas: "The recovery that was achieved can be explained very well by our established, natural neurophysiological processes, even if these neurological mechanisms remain misunderstood by the great majority of people. How could it be otherwise? Can you imagine that I was never taught, during all of my studies, what an emotion is! At medical school, we were never taught that body and mind are connected, that there is a complex network of communications between muscles and emotions, thoughts and immune system. Even if, in Phakyab Rinpoche's case, what happened is not common but exceptional, some hypotheses can be made. He might have triggered within himself the means to heal when his condition was beyond the normal or usual capacities for the body to heal. It is true that, normally, I can cure myself of some millions of germs in a wound, and yet it is beyond my reach if there are billions, and more so if there is a particularly virulent germ that overwhelms my defenses."

At Bellevue Hospital, I met one of the doctors who treated Rinpoche. He claimed that antibiotics had saved him. Rinpoche is convinced of the contrary. He had suffered side effects from the antibiotic treatment that disrupted his entire metabolism; it caused hypothyroidism, serious hepatitis, and severe gastric troubles. On a subtle level, this medication had gone so far as to affect the circulation of winds, and Rinpoche had to correct this imbalance with his meditative practice. I ask Dr. Coudron if Rinpoche could have benefited from the antibiotic treatment. "Maybe," he answers, "but it is not sure at all. What we know is that gangrene occurs, in the aftermath of wounds, because of an infection. An antibiotic treatment, in general, is not enough to check gangrene. It has to be accompanied by a local treatment to 'cleanse' the wound while a surgeon removes the necrotized — or dead — parts."

He continues, "That is why Rinpoche required amputation in view of the 'irreversible' destruction, according to medical reports. They were faced with serious gangrene, since there were foul smells that indicated a constant, evolving putrefaction of tissues, as well as a complete, in-depth destruction of the tissues of the joint, which was obvious on the X-rays. Usually, though it can be slowed thanks to antibiotics, such an illness leads to the death of the patient by septicemia. The prescription for Augmentin mentioned in his medical report was unfortunately ineffective, which explains the worsening of his condition. That is why they proposed amputation. Once Rinpoche refused it, from that moment on, the doctors only treated his pleurisy and his bone tuberculosis. They ceased to take responsibility for his gangrene. It is necessary to understand that it took two different steps to reach full recovery: on the one hand, stopping the infection, and on the other hand, reconstructing the ankle! This means that, even if the antibiotics prescribed for the tuberculosis had made the infection recede — which was not the case — they in no way could have been responsible for the reconstruction of tissues. This is why we can assert that it was not the antibiotic treatment that allowed healing. What enabled Rinpoche to heal was really his intensive work in meditation."

I ask Dr. Coudron about the links between the body's chemistry, the physical mechanisms of immunity, and the mind. In Rinpoche's case, a kind of nonphysical energy maximized the potential of his defenses and mobilized the resources of his body, which had remained inefficient for several months. How can it be explained, from a medical point of view, that Rinpoche managed to revive his capacities to heal himself?

For Dr. Coudron, the answer can be found in the very content of the practices, in which *tong-len* leads to the practice of *tsa-lung*. He says, "In circumstances like this one, when the mind is filled with altruistic love, kindness, and generosity, the body is in an optimal state to function. All the body flows are potentiated in a positive dynamic. When we can stay permanently in this state, through the practice of meditation, then we are ready."

The *tsa-lung* system was, for Dr. Coudron, an accelerator of the healing process that was engaged by meditation focused on compassion. He explains: "*Tsa-lung* is based on relaunching the flow of subtle winds in the body. When we suffer, there are blocks. Through visualization, and a benevolent attention to our body by focusing on the places where illness appears, we very clearly induce a real physiological action. By visualizing positively how our body functions, our brain and our body are in motion to allow it to heal. *Tong-len* enables a person to be in the best possible disposition, and *tsa-lung* directs, as a laser would, the necessary energy. The body then secretes what it needs to heal. Though it concerns the mind, meditation can only be effective if it is fully incarnated in the physical body. Such meditative states are by nature, for ordinary mortals, fleeting and transient, hard to implement in everyday life as long as the mind has not been stabilized. Hence Phakyab Rinpoche's reservations and desire to transmit the practices of *tsa-lung* only to practitioners he has specially trained. Thanks to his training, and to his exceptional personal aptitudes, he was able to mobilize the resources of his body and his mind to achieve what the New York doctors had deemed impossible, since they had all — with no exception — recommended amputation!"

I remark that *tsa-lung* is not well known by most people,

whereas compassion meditation, based on opening the heart, is within reach of the great majority of people. And its effects are no less therapeutic. Dr. Coudron agrees: "Compassion meditation puts the body in a state that maximizes all of its defenses and adaptive resources, contributing to optimal dynamics. By practicing *tong-len* several hours a day, Rinpoche enabled his body to permanently remain at the full capacity of his ability to heal. Admittedly, this does not mean that everyone suffering from tuberculosis or gangrene can heal thanks to meditation. For Rinpoche, it was the case. It is not a matter of chance that his wound, his infections, and his necrosis were suddenly able to evolve in the right direction. It is the result of an intense and very uncommon practice."

Dr. Coudron explains how, thanks to the state brought about by meditating on compassion, the immune defense system and white corpuscles multiplied. Armies of leukocytes, or white blood cells, eliminated the germs that were maintaining the infection and evacuated the dead cells. The leukocytes cleaned up the crumbled bits of cartilage, the necrotized fragments of bones, and all the useless tissues. This is what they do when, for example, they resorb the tip of a persistent herniated disc, the pus of an abscess, or the dead tissues of a bone. He says, "All this ability to heal is there, in our body. Rinpoche's state of unconditional compassion optimized them!"

Scientific Studies on the Therapeutic Power of Compassion

I try to understand what remained incomprehensible for the doctors at Bellevue Hospital in Rinpoche's recovery. I ask Dr. Coudron, "Aside from conventional treatments, how can one explain that, through compassion, the talus and tibial plafond — destroyed by septic arthritis — were able to regenerate? It normally takes no less than a bone transplant to achieve such a result. What link do you think there is between the practice of *tong-len,* associated with that of *tsa-lung,* and the regeneration of cartilage? And this happened precisely when medicine was expecting a more and more extensive necrosis together with a generalized septicemia?"

Dr. Coudron suggests a possible effect of practicing compassion meditation on a medical level, one that fits into our contemporary understanding of immunity: "By putting one's body in optimal conditions through *tong-len* meditation, and by concentrating all of one's energy onto the area that needs it through *tsa-lung* meditation, Phakyab Rinpoche gave the stem cells in his tissues, cartilage, and bones the capacity to reproduce themselves and to reform what he needed. In each cell of our body exist all the units of our body. Admittedly, Rinpoche did not reconstruct a brand new ankle, but a new functional 'neo-joint.' Genetic inheritance, in the form of strands of DNA, codifies all the cells in the chromosomes. For each cell, only one fraction of the unit is used, though all the units exist within the nucleus. Each part — corresponding to the tissue the cell is meant to be — expresses itself through a game of stop and go. The useless genes are blocked. If it is the bone, the part that codes genes for bones will express itself. Normally, only stem cells have the power to differentiate into any other cell. In theory, reforming affected parts of our body is possible, through this stop-and-go mechanism, except that we do not know how to really do it."

Dr. Coudron pauses, and with great humility and some perplexity, he explains that this phenomenon goes beyond contemporary medical knowledge: "That is actually where the miracle took place because, in actual fact, it is not possible. Something unusual happened, something that allowed Phakyab Rinpoche's cells to fight more efficiently against terribly aggressive germs, all while transforming stem cells to differentiate them into bone and cartilage. He therefore reconstructed his necrotized ankle.... This unusual something that happened was his meditation."

After some minutes of silence, Dr. Coudron continues. He insists that we possess an ability to self-heal, but it's necessary to create good conditions for that. The body must be in a state of peace and inner joy. As a practitioner, he sometimes uses therapies that stimulate the patient's own inner healing without any outside prescriptions. He says, "Whether it is acupuncture, psychotherapy, yoga, meditation — these methods never require any outside means. They mobilize our inner resources to trigger healing, which is in fact only our normal state! I therefore put my patients in the best possible conditions for their body and mind to better express themselves and release their healing potential. To help, I offer advice on respecting rhythms, healthy lifestyle, and food hygiene, as any doctor does his best to do. This is how, by mobilizing inner solutions, I see people living normally again after having been blocked for years by post-traumatic stress disorder. I notice that sleep becomes normal again, knee pain from terrible arthritis becomes painless. To me, these are little miracles of life that are reassuring examples of the exceptional means at our disposal in the heart of our flesh and of our soul. We thus live the miracle of our life in our lives."

The best therapy, according to Dr. Coudron, and the process that triggers self-healing, remains undoubtedly meditation on compassion. Meditation training like this is accessible to all, and it increases our capacity to trust ourselves, whether we are beginners or advanced meditators.

"That does not mean, and I insist on this point," Dr. Coudron warns, "that we give up all medical solutions, that we put aside chemotherapy in case of cancer, that we stop taking our anti-angina medication in case of myocardial ischemia, that we give up neuroleptics if we need them. Rather, we should just continue to develop within what enables us to be at our best in all circumstances. If Phakyab Rinpoche was able to heal, this means that, following his example, it is up to us to develop our means of healing. Even if we cannot necessarily do what he accomplished, he shows us the way and inspires us to surpass ourselves and better our lives. Meditating is within everyone's reach. This is all the more important for two reasons, as his positive example shows. It not only helps the one who practices meditation, but it encourages developing better relations with others, which leads to exceptional happiness. The path is more important than the goal. If we take this path of inner transformation, both we ourselves and those around us will benefit from it."

During our talk, Dr. Coudron expresses genuine joy. Yet afterward, he continues examining Phakyab Rinpoche's medical files, and in the days that follow, he sends me a written report of astonishing depth. He notes the peculiarity of Rinpoche's healing and the strength of his methods. The report reads, in part: "Despite myself, by virtue of my scientific medical training, I could not help looking for a flaw, but to no avail. Was there something the doctors hadn't seen, or was his condition not so catastrophic? But no, everything was clear, nothing wrong about it. Phakyab Rinpoche had really been admitted in the hospital...in May 2003 and had left it after...six months, on his own initiative, truly refusing the operation they were suggesting. The checkups really show there was a major risk, that his joint was irreversibly destroyed. Without amputation, it was life-threatening."

Dr. Coudron also reviews the latest X-ray reports. Yes, there has been a healing, and it goes against all the initial medical hypotheses. Today, Phakyab Rinpoche is fine, and he still has his two legs. He walks like before, and the examinations show that everything has been sufficiently reconstructed to enable him to live a normal life.

To understand the full mechanisms of his healing, one undoubtedly needs to be schooled by compassion, as it is taught in particular by Tibetan lamas. However, scientific studies on compassion have shown the same thing. In particular, one study was published in 2013 by Steven Cole, a professor of medicine at the University of California at Los Angeles, and his colleagues. He demonstrated that benevolence, more than any other emotion, has a positive effect on the immune system. As Dr. Coudron described, each cell in our body contains all twenty-one thousand genes of our genetic code, but depending on each cell's function, some genes will be repressed, meaning they do not express themselves, while others do express themselves. Certain emotions or conditions also affect the expression of genes. We know that stress encourages the expression of genes that lead to illness, whereas happiness allows the expression of genes that facilitate the good functioning of our body. In his study, Steven Cole showed that the cause of our happiness also has an effect. He distinguished *hedonic* happiness, or the immediate pleasure one feels from satisfying one's desires, from *eudaimonic* happiness, or the pleasure one feels by acting benevolently or compassionately toward others. According to this study, experiencing hedonic happiness or pleasure, similar to stress, leads to an increase of proinflammatory symptoms and a decrease of antiviral activity and antibodies! One would think that getting what you want would improve your health, but according to Steven Cole, this is not the case, and it even seems to be detrimental! Meanwhile, experiencing eudaimonic happiness leads to a slightly increased expression of anti-inflammatory genes and a strong expression of antiviral genes, which allow the creation of antibodies.

Steven Cole concluded: "What this study shows us is that doing good and feeling good have very different effects on the genome. Even if they generate similar levels of positive emotions, it seems that the human genome is much more sensitive to the means used to reach this happiness than our mind is."

A few days later, responding to the results of this study, Dr. Coudron tells me: "That is exactly what I retain from Phakyab Rinpoche's teaching. It is what the story of his healing shows. It takes all its meaning in the dimension of unconditional compassion."

Healing and Contemplative Neurosciences

Phakyab Rinpoche is aware that his story, and the increasingly documented positive effects of compassion, can lead to a different problem, that of unrealistic expectations. People come to see him hoping for a miraculous healing, but everyone is different. Rinpoche always encourages people to follow their medical protocols, and he often mentions the case of one of his students in California. He had urged her not to rely only on meditation to cure her advanced-stage cancer. He knew she was not experienced or proficient enough as a meditator to do so. She did not listen to him, and he was sad when her health inexorably deteriorated.

It would be wrong to interpret Phakyab Rinpoche's testimony as encouraging people to give up all medical care or to completely rely on spiritual practice for healing. As Rinpoche often recalls, the published research studies in contemplative neurosciences — which concluded that cerebral plasticity enables us to train and physically modify the brain — involved very experienced meditators, people who had accomplished between ten thousand and fifty thousand hours of meditation devoted to developing compassion, altruism, attention, and mindfulness.

Experienced meditators show an exceptional capacity to voluntarily create and maintain precise, powerful, and durable mental states. These states can be spotted in certain well-identified areas of the brain, and they are only reached with mental training. Just like an athlete, one's skill and achievements correlate to the number of hours of practice. As of 2014, Rinpoche had accomplished almost eighty thousand hours of meditation, which is much more than the meditators used in the studies. Furthermore, the three-year curriculum that Rinpoche has created in healing sciences and inner yoga includes quantifying the hours of practice. Meditators are asked to take note of, day after day, the number of hours spent on the cushion. Admittedly, reaching a certain number does not guarantee the quality of awakened mindfulness that someone will be able to generate, but nothing is possible without regular training. It is a decisive criterion of progression.

Medicine, an Art of Giving

The discoveries in contemplative neurosciences are encouraging. In these studies, the essential dimension of altruism has been added, and it's been shown that, even without being a highly trained meditator, one can benefit from the positive effects of meditation centered on love and compassion. For example, twenty minutes a day can reduce anxiety and stress, and for those with serious depression, it can lower the risk of having a relapse. If the brain is regularly stimulated, some thirty days is enough to bring about changes in neuronal functions.

"Phakyab Rinpoche's testimony concerns all of us," Dr. Coudron insists. "Despite its exceptional and spectacular character, it is accessible to most of us, even if we haven't been trained in meditation as much as he has. And the methods he teaches can perfectly support a treatment. They allow us to take advantage of a treatment's utmost benefits while neutralizing the undesirable side effects."

I ask Dr. Coudron if, one day, there is a chance that medical knowledge and the inner sciences of healing, which Phakyab Rinpoche is teaching in France, will come together. Dr. Coudron is positive they will. He says, "For care teams, complementarities between medicine and meditation are of course possible, in accordance with Phakyab Rinpoche's wish. Contemporary studies are going in that direction, and the therapeutic benefits of meditation are better and better known. The Medical School at the University of Strasbourg, on Dr. Jean-Gérard Bloch's initiative, even offers a university degree entitled 'Medicine, Meditation, and Neurosciences.'"

I tell Dr. Coudron that Phakyab Rinpoche and I have met Dr. Jean-Gérard Bloch ourselves in Strasbourg. Along with psychiatrist Dr. Gilles Bertschy, Dr. Bloch runs a training program for psychologists and researchers in the neurosciences that merges meditation with theoretical reflection. Intended for health care professionals, the program tackles such subjects as consciousness, the nature of the mind, and the link between body and mind, and the interdisciplinary curriculum includes philosophy, history of medicine, psychology, psychiatry, endocrinology, and immunology.

"Approaching meditation in this way, within the academic, institutional framework of the medical school," Dr. Bloch explained to us, "vouches for the growing interest nowadays in a knowledge based on the experience of body-mind interaction. Within the framework of health care medicine, there is no question of replacing Western medicine with meditation, but rather of associating them, so that their potential may maximize each other in a holistic approach of integrative medicine."

Dr. Bloch spoke with a certain reserve, in which I perceived great open-mindedness and great respect for others. He did not seek to impose his ideas. This is a sign of maturity in the practice of meditation, and I asked who he had trained with. I was moved when he mentioned Tarab Rinpoche, and I felt through him the presence of this spiritual master who inspires him. An accomplished meditator of dream yoga — and thus able to follow the mysterious paths taken by consciousness during sleep — as well as an erudite philosopher and master in Buddhist dialectics, Tarab Rinpoche was invited to come teach in Denmark in 1962 by Prince Peter of Greece and Denmark.

For more than thirty years, as a researcher and lecturer at Copenhagen University and at the Royal Library, Tarab Rinpoche developed a universal school of thought based on the paradigm of interdependence, the keystone of Buddhist wisdom. His education program, entitled "Unity in Duality," matched, according to Dr. Bloch, the scientific developments that had become available for thirty years in the field of contemplative neurosciences. But the person who first truly integrated meditation with science and medicine was Professor Jon Kabat-Zinn. In 1979, he founded the Mindfulness-Based Stress Reduction program at the University of Massachusetts Medical School, which today is a basis for the University of Strasbourg's degree in Medicine, Meditation, and Neurosciences.

Dr. Lionel Coudron agrees with Dr. Bloch that research studies are multiplying nowadays, and they examine not only changes in physiology resulting from meditation but also the various health benefits. He says, "It is gradual and slow work still, even if we sometimes have the feeling of making giant steps. I am certain that this book will contribute to making things much more dynamic, and that it will subsequently bring a wider audience. This testimony adds a building block to the issue, and it demonstrates the interest it arouses today."

To free our inner resources, we have simple methods at our disposal that are easy to access and accomplish. Phakyab Rinpoche invites us to transform our mind without waiting to be ill, and especially without rejecting anything offered by modern medicine.

He proves to us, in a very convincing way, that meditating on compassion is a path toward healing.

I agree with Dr. Coudron that Rinpoche's exemplary benevolence and forgiveness toward his torturers, and his loving mind, which emerged triumphant over gangrene and bone tuberculosis, encourage us to develop more kindness in our everyday life. By drawing inspiration from him, we can have a healthier, sounder, and happier life, for ourselves and for everyone close to us. Healing physical illness can be a step toward ultimate healing, toward the great Awakening.

During our conversations, Dr. Coudron sat in his office under a depiction of Sangye Menla, the Tibetan Medicine Buddha, surrounded by his manifestations, the seven Medicine Buddhas who work to relieve the sufferings of all living beings. His words on compassion, and his benevolent attitude, resonate with the teachings of Kalu Rinpoche, a great master for whom the art of healing is the art of giving and verges on the sacred:

> If two doctors, one in a spirit of compassion, the other not, give the same medicine, the one given by the first will be more efficient than the one given by the second. This is only because the treatment will also be full of the strength of love and compassion, a very great strength....
>
> In India, there was a very wise man called Atisha. He came to Tibet to give rise to a new development of Buddhist teachings.
>
> One day, Atisha had an illness on his hand. He had a disciple whose name was Dromteunpa. He was only a simple, faithful layman, but he was a very close disciple.
>
> Atisha asked him to take his hand in his and to blow on it. Dromteunpa answered: "Certainly not, I have no power, and nothing at all will happen."
>
> Atisha told him: "Yes, because you have much love,

much compassion, and therefore I am sure that if you hold my hand in yours, and you blow on it, it will be cured."

Dromteunpa then blew on it, and Atisha's illness was cured.

EPILOGUE

In This Life and in All Lives

I Will Be Completely Healed
When You Finish Writing This Book

July 21, 2014. We are approaching Dharamsala, where Rinpoche wanted to be as we finish this book.

The morning sky is heavy under the screen of monsoon clouds, which veil the sun and temper the heat. The steep road suddenly reveals the heights of the Dhauladhar range, dominated by wide sections of black granite and gray slate and crowned by everlasting snow. Halfway down the slope, there are hanging banks of rhododendron and oleanders and ravines of bougainvillea. Then, as we ascend, I joyfully hail the first Himalayan cedars. Throughout history, the *devadaru* or deodars — which means "trees of God" — have sheltered the long ascetic periods of wise men, offering them their subtle fragrances as incense to open the doors to spiritual levels. Their trunks, covered with large sepia scales and bordered with black rings, ascend high into the sky.

The thin asphalt ribbon continues to wind up the slope of a rocky spur. Twin hills, nestled in a thick forest, stand out. The first bears the buildings of Namgyal, the Dalai Lama's private monastery, and the second one bears his residence, perched like the nest of an eagle. The conversation with Rinpoche has been lively since we left the Kangra Valley and the former Maharaja city with its splendors and legendary palaces. As we approach the places where Kundun went into exile fifty years earlier, we become silent. Rinpoche collects himself. Telling his *mala*, he whispers the Avalokiteshvara mantra as we enter the Tibetan colony of Dharamsala.

The Himalayan town is now completely overcome by the speculative fever of Indian businessmen. It even affects the outskirts of Namgyal Monastery, which once remained preserved. On the construction sites of buildings — which have become higher and higher and more and more numerous — Indian women grown old before their time and scraggly children carry bricks, gravel, and sand in laden baskets on their heads. The construction of new hotels, restaurants, and shops is intended to welcome the crowds that have become heavier in recent years. People flow in from all over the world for teaching sessions, and they crowd by the thousands around the Dalai Lama. As he tries to enlighten them, rather than convert them, he inspires their existential quest and helps create the causes of happiness by developing inner peace.

Yellow-and-black taxis and power-driven rickshaws jostle one another and sound their horns along the single road stretching along the slopes.

"We even manage to have traffic jams. Isn't that a criterion of development?" says Samdhong Rinpoche* amusingly, with a mischievous gleam in his solemn and benevolent eyes.

---

* Samdhong Rinpoche has been the Dalai Lama's companion in exile since 1959, and he was close to Jiddu Krishnamurti. He was the prime minister of the Tibetan government in exile from 2001 to 2011 and spokesman of Satyagraha following the Mahatma Gandhi.

Despite the arrival of modernity in Dharamsala, I can still find the same vibration of consciousness in Namgyal Temple, unchanged, powerful, and liberating. The local animals are steeped in it, such as the eagles, hawks, and crows that tirelessly circle in wide sweeps above Kundun's residence. Or like the temple's many hieratic dogs that sit for long hours near the monks. With a peaceful gentleness and cat-like calmness, they do not bark by day. But as soon as night shrouds the heights, and the cicadas chirp rapturously, they start their endless chatting through the valley — would they have understood, in their own way, the art of debate that monks practice with such zeal?

At dawn on the second day in Dharamsala, which rises in an exultation of golden and crimson shades, I recall Rinpoche's words, twice repeated. The first time was when he asked me to write the story of his healing, and then again in New York six months ago: "I will be completely healed when you finish writing this book."

Completely healed? What exactly does he mean? The answer comes at the end of our stay in Dharamsala.

We sit on a bench along the Lingkor, the ritual circumambulation path winding around Kundun's residence, and we overlook the Kangra Valley as far as the eye can see. The path is bordered with devotion flags hanging from the treetops and prayer wheels that turn and ring a bronze bell. Tibetans of all ages walk up and down this road to receive the blessings of their charismatic leader, while the deep voices of the monastic college of Namgyal resonate, with cymbals, drums, horns, and bone flutes. It is the sixth lunar month, and the monks are performing the great Chakrasamvara ritual. They are creating its sand-colored mandala, which is the basis of the *tsa-lung* practice that allowed Rinpoche to heal. Finishing the book here makes sense. We are back where it all started.

For a new start.

"I have three great missions in this life," Rinpoche tells me, looking introspective. "First, as a human being. Second, as a teacher of Dharma. Third, as a lama, holder of a lineage. As a human being, at the age of thirteen, I offered my life to the service of all beings. In my experience of the world, I have therefore adopted an open-minded, trustful, and spontaneously welcoming attitude toward all those who cross my path through maturation of karma. Nobody I meet is foreign to me. In each one, I find my brothers and sisters in humanity. As human beings, we all have within us the jewel of awakened mind, which is our extraordinary potential for kindness and inner transformation.

"At the basis of my teachings, there is the opening of the heart, and I endeavor to introduce my students into the mind's spacious states, which encompass the universes and all beings. Meditating on the opening of the heart concerns everyone, Buddhists as well as non-Buddhists, for it nurtures the fundamental human values of love, benevolence, compassion, forgiveness, human rights, and reconciliation. Without an opening of the heart, our ethics remain unembodied and can very well veer toward intolerance. Taking the path of the heart always helps us recognize the potential for kindness and transformation that is a feature of our humanity. If we have developed unconditional love, we will recognize this loving basis even in the cruelest among us, who act inhumanly because they ignore their true nature. Opening the heart makes us love beings so much that every day we renew our ever-keener longing to help them, so that they may find happiness and be delivered from suffering.

"In my efforts to relieve the sufferings of the world, I feel particularly concerned by the fate of mothers who die while giving life. This happened with my sister when, at the age of twenty-six, she gave birth to my nephew. Just like her, for lack of means, many other mothers in remote areas of Tibet, or in the Tibetan colonies in India, are not granted the care they need to survive childbirth, and so raise their children. It is a double misfortune, the misfortune of the mother and the misfortune of the little orphans. My first mission in this life is therefore to teach a code of ethics of the heart and to implement a humanitarian program that cares for future mothers and helps educate their children, in particular girls. It is essential that the most destitute girl should be able to access higher education and be granted an equal status with men. 'When a woman is educated, a people is educated,' such is a saying of traditional wisdom. Women are the key to evolution and to a better future for humanity."

The Medicine Buddha, among his twelve great vows, promised to help women who have the particular karma of giving life after much suffering. He also committed himself to lead them on the path of perfect Awakening. I am moved to hear that the first mission of Phakyab Rinpoche is in line with this aspiration, as he places the power of his compassionate action in the service of mothers and their children.

Rinpoche continues, "As a master of Dharma, I have a second mission. It is also in the realm of suffering, not suffering on a relative level this time, but on an ultimate level, the very causes of suffering. The root cause of all our pains is fundamental ignorance. Our erroneous understanding of reality maintains destructive states of mind, such as hatred, attachment, desire, jealousy, and anger. These emotions carry on the cycle of suffering and make us turn our backs on happiness. My mission is therefore to unceasingly provide the teachings that deliver us from ignorance by conquering our inner enemies. Believing in adversity is a terrible illusion. The enemies that appear outside of us are the projections of our uncontrolled mind. When we have overcome all our inner demons, nothing can affect us anymore.

"The Buddha's life offers several examples of the perfectly

mastered power of the mind. One day, out of jealousy, his cousin Devadatta launched against him one of the most ferocious elephants, thinking the animal would pierce him with his tusks or trample him. But as it approached the Awakened, the elephant knelt down. Then, on the night of the Buddha's Awakening, the demon of death, Mara, sent the anger of the winds against the great meditator. But though their fury could uproot trees, the winds did not crumple a fold of his robe. Mara then called forth torrential rains, which racked the earth. They did not wet a single fiber of the Buddha's clothes. And when, in the end, Mara ordered his troops to destroy the Awakened, the arrows became flowers at the touch of his body. The light radiating from him was like a shield protecting him, so that the swords were broken, and the axes were nicked. Such is the power of the mind when established in primordial peace. With my training, since my first years at Golok Monastery, and with the experience of my remarkable healing, I must now especially teach inner peace, which reveals the mind's boundless power of healing. If possible, I want to encourage therapists and doctors to integrate the spiritual dimension of human beings into their understanding of illness and care giving. This is my second mission as a teacher of Dharma, since my healing, to be complete, must be dedicated to the ultimate healing of all lives. I have vowed to heal in the name of all beings. This vow is being fulfilled, Sofia, with the testimony of this book. I have shared this life experience with you in order to help my readers better recognize the power of their own mind."

These words of Phakyab Rinpoche resonate like the call of a guru from the heart of compassion. They wrap us in a powerful vibration that reaches from era to era, and echoes through the memory of worlds, in this life and in all lives.

"And at last," Rinpoche says, "I have a third mission, as the holder of a lineage. Acknowledged as the eighth Phakyab

Rinpoche, I must preserve a spiritual filiation and carry on the memory of my lineage, of these extraordinary teachers who made the offerings of all their lives to all beings before me. For I am the holder of the throne of Ashi Monastery, blessed by the heart relics of Je Tsongkhapa, which some Tibetans saved from destruction by the Red Guards at the peril of their lives. In the past few years, thanks to the generosity of my students, I have been able to rebuild Je Tsongkhapa's chapel, and soon I hope to be able to set up a patronage program to ensure a sufficient amount of daily food for the monks of Ashi."

It is unthinkable for Rinpoche to fail his duty as safeguard of the sacred heritage of his lineage, no less precious than his own life. I am moved as he mentions his spiritual inheritance in front of the residence of the Dalai Lama, who, in the inextricable nebula of karmic causes and effects, acknowledged him twenty years earlier as the eighth reincarnation of a great lineage.

We lift up our heads to the rustle of wings. A hawk flies in circles over us. Is it here to seal Rinpoche's words with the stamp of promise, the promise that he will unfailingly achieve the three great missions of his life?

"Thank you, Sofia, for having written my story," Phakyab Rinpoche says. "I am thus totally healed because everything, everything has been put into action. With this book, and in accordance with Kundun's message, which I received eleven years ago on my hospital bed, the time has come for me to teach the world how to heal."

Chronology of
Phakyab Rinpoche's Healing

Excerpts from the medical reports of consultations
at Bellevue Hospital in Manhattan

2003

May 23

RADIOLOGY DEPARTMENT

There is generalized osteopenia.

There is marked bone resorption and fragmentation at the ankle joint, involving the tibial plafond and talar dome suspicious for septic arthritis. The tarsal bones are not well visualized, and appear largely fused.

Findings suspicious for septic arthritis of the ankle joint; fusion of the intertarsal joints noted.

June 4

ORTHOPEDICS DEPARTMENT

Right ankle pain/swelling and purulent discharge of 4 weeks duration, and X-ray picture of infectious arthritis with destruction of ankle joint. Patient was advised Below Knee Amputation but he refused and he is currently on Augmentin, NWB [non-weight-bearing] with crutches.

June 12

INFECTIOUS DISEASE DEPARTMENT

No fever, no generalized infection.

Right ankle fracture several years ago. Necrotic bone but patient refused BKA [below knee amputation]. Still on Augmentin (for approximately 2 weeks). Patient has purulence on both sides of ankle, demonstrating that a deep bone infection exists. Patient requests continuing antibiotics rather than surgery, despite the need for surgery. Will therefore continue Augmentin, and monitor patient, who is also followed by orthopedics.

June 17

PROGRAM FOR SURVIVORS OF TORTURE —
ADMISSIONS INTERVIEW

July 24

VIROLOGY DEPARTMENT

Patient not interested in amputation and has therefore been placed on long-term Augmentin until worsens or agrees to amputation.

I have discussed in detail patient's prognosis and likely course.

September 13

RADIOLOGY DEPARTMENT

No evidence of deep veinous thrombosis.
Marked atrophy of right thigh muscles.

September 14

RADIOLOGY DEPARTMENT

Right pleural effusion. Paraspinal abscess.

September 17
RADIOLOGY DEPARTMENT

Right foot and ankle: patient has complete disruption of the tibiotalar joint with almost complete loss of the talus. There is soft tissue swelling in the region. Osteomyelitis cannot be ruled out in the region.

There is diffuse arthritic changes about the tarsic region involving all joints.

September 19
RADIOLOGY DEPARTMENT

Infective Pleural Effusion.

September 20
RADIOLOGY DEPARTMENT

Generalized osteopenia. There is persistent marked bone resorption and fragmentation at the ankle joint, with involvement of the tibial plafond and talar dome. Findings suggest osteomyelitis, and a septic joint.

September 22
CYTOLOGY REPORT

Paraspinal fluid collection.
Lymphocytic predominant exudative pleural effusion.

October 6
MEDICINE CLINIC — AMBCARE NOTE

Increasing SOB [shortness of breath], pluiritic chest pain. Also ankle is hurting with increased drainage. (Tylenol warm compresses).

Pleuritis and back pain, found with paraspinal abscess, and exudative pleural effusion. Plural biopsy with granulomas.

Right ankle with ++ swelling.

Back pain from compression of nerve from Pott's disease.

October 14
ORTHOPEDICS DEPARTMENT

X-rays: completely destroyed ankle joint. Patient with chronic infection of right foot and ankle.

Will refer patient to Physical Therapist to see other patients with below knee amputation and prostheses.

Ortho clinic and previous consultations recommended below knee amputation as debridement of foot would leave a nonviable ankle joint and foot.

October 22
ORTHOPEDICS DEPARTMENT

Pott's disease, tuberculosis, pleuritis.

Here with victims of torture translator/social worker. Very concerned about right ankle chronic destructive arthritis. Orthopedist wants to amputate — not enough viable tissue to either heal or save.

Discussed at length possibility that prosthesis would work.

Patient needs below knee amputation, but would like to see more tuberculosis treatment before final decision.

November 26
CHEST — AMBCARE NOTE

Patient saw outside orthopedist. Since ankle is destroyed and issue of infection would be difficult to put aside (recurrent infection possible), possibilities for reconstruction very limited and amputation would probably yield best functional outcome.

December 15
MEDICINE CLINIC — AMBCARE NOTE

Diabetes, Type II N
Tuberculosis of Vertebra
Anemia
Abnormal Liver Function

2004

January 21
RADIOLOGY DEPARTMENT

Lucency and periostitis in the region of the right medial malleolus appears to have healed somewhat since the previous study of 9/20/03; moreover the overall bone density appears more uniform and there has been interval resolution of some of the mottled osteopenia noted on the earlier examination.

Impression: Chronic destructive arthritis of the right ankle joint, consistent with the clinical diagnosis of septic arthritis.

July 7
CHEST — AMBCARE NOTE

Right ankle much improved, no pain. Able to walk without crutches most of time.

September 8
CHEST — AMBCARE NOTE

Right ankle still improving. No pain. Able to walk without crutches most of time.

September 29

CHEST — AMBCARE NOTE

Right ankle still improving. No pain. Able to walk without crutches most of time.

Will get orthosis follow up after ankle is optimized.

Getting better all the time.

Epigastric burning.

December 29

CHEST — AMBCARE NOTE

Right ankle much better. No pain. Able to walk without crutches most of time.

2005

February 16

CHEST — AMBCARE NOTE

Right ankle getting better and better. No pain. Able to walk 2 or 3 blocks without crutches, before stopping because of pain.

March 30

CHEST — AMBCARE NOTE

Right ankle getting better and better. No pain. Able to walk 2 or 3 blocks without crutches, before stopping because of pain.

April 8

CHEST — AMBCARE NOTE

Spinal tuberculosis healed.

April 20
RADIOLOGY DEPARTMENT

Pictures of right ankle show irregular aspect of articular margin of lower tibia, as well as an erosion of the posterior foot bone, including the talus, the calcaneus, and some bones of the tarsus. There are irregularities in the other parts of the talus, and fragmentation in some areas.

June 16
MEDICINE CLINIC — AMBCARE NOTE

End of two years of multiple antibiotic treatments.

September 6
MEDICINE CLINIC — AMBCARE NOTE

Patient now walks up to five blocks but is limited by pain on right ankle. He can stand without significant pain for two hours. Wound well healed.

September 30
MEDICINE CLINIC — AMBCARE NOTE

The volume of destruction of the central bone in the intradiscal zone has slightly diminished. Observations in coherence with the progressive healing of the spine tuberculosis.

December 27
BRACE AMBCARE NOTE

Patient able to walk 10 city blocks with one crutch.
Patient fitted for solid AFO [ankle foot orthosis].

2006

January 9

MEDICINE CLINIC — AMBCARE NOTE

Marked improvement in ambulation.

1 week before stopping tuberculosis medication, patient reported noting a little blood in vomit.

2009

February 9

MEDICINE CLINIC — AMBCARE NOTE

Patient has been walking without any problem for over a year.

2013

January 28

MEDICINE CLINIC — AMBCARE NOTE

Old scarring, well healed from prior gangrene.

2014

November 4

REPORT ON X-RAY OF RIGHT ANKLE REQUESTED BY DR. COUDRON

Osteo-necrosis of the talar dome, the tibial plafond and the lower part of the tibia.

A new-joint has been created between the tibia and what is left of the talus. The calcaneum seems normal.

ENDNOTES

———◆·◇·◆———

BOOK ONE

Chapter One: I Grew Up with Growing Mountains

Page 11, *As a star, a hallucination, the flame of a lamp:* This quote is from the original French edition of this book; it is a new English translation for this edition.

Page 13, *Even if the Buddha is not present:* This quote is from the original French edition of this book; it is a new English translation for this edition.

Page 26, *May all sentient beings enjoy happiness, and the causes of happiness:* This traditional Buddhist prayer is known as the "Four Immeasurables." This version is from the original French edition of this book; it is a new English translation for this edition.

Page 29, *Have you received the teaching of a wise master:* This excerpt is adapted from Alexandra David-Neel, *Immortality and Reincarnation: Wisdom from the Forbidden Journey*, trans. Jon Graham (Rochester, VT: Inner Traditions International, 1997).

Chapter Two: Ragged Yak

Page 42, *I am a sage who possesses in plentitude the manifold treasures of desire:* Ronald Herder, ed., *Songs of Milarepa* (Mineola, NY: Dover Thrift Editions, Dover Publications, 2003).

Chapter Three: Night of Pain in Tibet

Page 47, *Now as long as space endures:* Shantideva, *The Way of the Bodhisattva (Bodhicaryvatara)*, rev. ed., trans. Padmakara Translation Group (1997, 2006; Boston and London: Shambhala Publications, 2011), ch. 10, verse 55.

Page 48, *This Earth, anointed with perfume, flowers strewn:* Thubten Chodron, *Cultivating a Compassionate Heart: The Yoga Method of Chenreẑig* (Ithaca, NY: Snow Lion Publications, 2005), 19.

Page 53, *When the iron bird flies:* This well-known quote is from the original French edition of this book; it is a new English translation for this edition.

Page 54, *He who, today, is my follower, the Lotus-Perfume monk:* This quote is a new English translation for this edition from Françoise Wang, *Djé Tsongkhapa* (Paris: Editions Détchène Eusèl Ling, 2000).

Chapter Four: The Program for Survivors of Torture

Page 79, *Om, homage to the Venerable Tara:* This traditional prayer to Tara is from the original French edition of this book; it is a new English translation for this edition.

Chapter Five: Cutting Is Not Curing: I Refuse Amputation

Page 104, *When I see beings of unpleasant character:* Geshe Langri Tangpa, "Eight Verses of Training the Mind," verse 4, English translation from Dalailama.com, http://dalailama.com/teachings/training-the-mind /verse-4.

Page 104, *This is the supreme draft of immortality:* Shantideva, *The Way of the Bodhisattva*, rev. ed., trans. Padmakara Translation Group (1997, 2006; Boston and London: Shambhala Publications, 2011), ch. 3, verses 29–32.

Chapter Six: Balancing My Happiness against the Suffering of Others

Page 115, *May I be a guard for those who are protectorless:* Shantideva, *The Way of the Bodhisattva*, rev. ed., trans. Padmakara Translation Group (1997,

2006; Boston and London: Shambhala Publications, 2011), ch. 3, verses 18–21.

Page 117, *May beings everywhere who suffer:* Shantideva, *The Way of the Bodhisattva*, rev. ed., trans. Padmakara Translation Group (1997, 2006; Boston and London: Shambhala Publications, 2011), ch. 10, verse 2.

Page 118, *All suffering without exception arises from desiring happiness for oneself:* Dilgo Khyentse, *The Heart of Compassion: The Thirty-Seven Verses on the Practice of a Bodhisattva*, trans. Padmakara Translation Group (Boston and London: Shambhala Publications, 2012), verse 11.

Page 118: *All the violence, all the perils, all the sufferings of the world:* This quote is from the original French edition of this book; it is a new English translation for this edition.

Page 119, *May beings everywhere who suffer:* Shantideva, *The Way of the Bodhisattva*, rev. ed., trans. Padmakara Translation Group (1997, 2006; Boston and London: Shambhala Publications, 2011), excerpts from ch. 10.

Chapter Seven:
Why Do You Seek Healing outside of Yourself?

Page 143, *You are quite mistaken, says the Blessed:* This quote is from the original French edition of this book; it is a new English translation for this edition.

Page 144, *That is why the Blessed claims to have reached Awakening:* Gautama Buddha, *The Lotus Sutra: Saddharma-Pundarika*, trans. H. Kern (CreateSpace Independent Publishing Platform, June 2015).

Page 148, *In this pure land surrounded by the snowy mountains:* This translation is available from the International Kalachakra Network, kalachakranet .org/teachings/long_life/LLhhdlr.rtf.

Chapter Eight: My Meditation Grotto in Brooklyn

Page 170, *In brief, may I offer benefit and joy:* Geshe Langri Tangpa, "Eight Verses of Training the Mind," verses 7 and 8, English translation from Dalailama.com, http://dalailama.com/teachings/training-the-mind.

Page 177, *Just as a mother would protect her only child at the risk of her own life:* Peter Harvey, *An Introduction to Buddhism: Teachings, History, and Practices* (New York: Cambridge University Press, 2012), 279.

BOOK TWO
Chapter One: The Sutra of the Heroic March

Page 200, *Clear light, that has its source within itself, and that was never born:* This quote is a new English translation of Gustave-Charles Toussaint, trans., *Padmasambhava: Le Dict de Padma* (Paris: Les Deux Océans, 2000).

Page 212, *Sofia, you wrote the Dalai Lama's* Spiritual Autobiography: The Dalai Lama and Sofia Stril-Rever, *My Spiritual Autobiography* (New York: HarperOne, 2010), and the Dalai Lama and Sofia Stril-Rever, *My Appeal to the World*, trans. Sebastian Houssiaux (New York: Tibet House, 2015).

Chapter Two: An Exceptionally Powerful Healing

Page 224, *In particular, one study was published in 2013 by Steven Cole:* Barbara Frederickson, et al., "A Functional Genomic Perspective on Human Well-Being," *Proceedings of the National Academy of Sciences* 110, no. 33 (August 13, 2013), doi: 10.1073/pnas.1305419110.

Page 225, *As Rinpoche often recalls, the published research studies*: A program based on research made, originally, by Francisco Varela in France, and carried on by Richard Davidson and Antoine Lutz in Madison, Paul Ekman and Robert Levenson in San Francisco and Berkeley, Jonathan Cohen and Brent Field at Princeton, Stephen Kosslyn at Harvard, and Tania Singer in Zurich, these names being only the best known, to which we could add Matthieu Ricard, who was operational in making the results of these studies widely known to the greater public, while actively taking part in them as a subject of experimentation.

Page 229, *If two doctors, one in a spirit of compassion, the other not:* This quote is a new English translation of Kalu Rinpoche, *Le Bouddha de la médecine et son mandala* (Marpa Editions, 1998).

Phakyab Rinpoche's Associations

Menla Thödöl Ling

In 2013, Phakyab Rinpoche and Sofia Stril-Rever cofounded Menla Thödöl Ling, "The Garden of Liberation through Listening to the Medicine Buddha," in the valley of the Eure River, near Paris. It is a sanctuary dedicated to natural life, inhabited by wild birds and swans. This is the Buddhist teaching center in which Phakyab Rinpoche first started teaching his nine-step path toward *shamatha*. This program, called "Experiencing Peace and Inner Healing," is a three-year cycle in which students build up a certain number of hours of practice to access its different stages. It prepares them for the *tsa-lung* practices, the inner winds yoga that allowed Rinpoche to heal. Five hundred people have already enrolled in the program. The curriculum is adapted to the Western way of life, led by a teaching staff, and adjusted according to the schedule of each individual. Additional information can be found at www.phakyabrinpoche.org.

Tibet Mother & Child International (TMCI)

Still in the planning stages, this program is being designed to address Phakyab Rinpoche's wish to help young Tibetan mothers who, both in their country and in exile in India, are not granted medical care during their pregnancy or after childbirth. Rinpoche also intends to support them by providing schooling for their children. For the time being, some help is being provided on a limited basis to Tibetan families who have asked Rinpoche for it.

Healing Buddha Foundation

The Healing Buddha Foundation seeks to help spread Phakyab Rinpoche's teachings around the world. It is a 501(c)(3) nonprofit organization established in the United States to encourage and enable the well-being and the development of people facing suffering of all types. The organization widely promotes the transmission of Buddhist inner sciences and ethics, while preserving the unique Tibetan cultural heritage. It empowers Tibetan refugee mothers and their children to become healthy, educated, and economically self-sustaining community members. And it supplements the operating expenses of the Ashi and Golok Monasteries in Tibet and the Sera Mey Monastery in India. Additional information can be found at http://healingbuddhafoundation.org.

Books by Sofia Stril-Rever

In addition to the books listed here, Sofia Stril-Rever has recorded the CD *Dakinis: Sacred Chants of Tibet* (Sometime Studio, October 2012), and she coauthored the film *Dalai Lama: Une vie après l'autre* [*Life After Life*] for the television channel Arte, which was broadcast worldwide on August 10, 2008.

Books Translated into English

My Appeal to the World. With the Dalai Lama (New York: Tibet House, 2015).
My Spiritual Journey. With the Dalai Lama (New York: HarperOne, 2010).

Books in French

Sœur Emmanuelle, mon amie, ma mère, with Sister Sara, Presses de la Renaissance, 2009
Mon testament spirituel de sœur Emmanuelle, Presses de la Renaissance, 2008
365 méditations de sœur Emmanuelle, Presses de la Renaissance, 2008
Kalachakra, Un mandala pour la paix, préface du Dalaï-lama, photographies de Matthieu Ricard, Manuel Bauer et Olivier Adam, La Martinière, 2008
Mille et un bonheurs, Méditations de sœur Emmanuelle, Carnets Nord, 2007
La Folie d'amour, Entretiens avec sœur Emmanuelle, J'ai lu 2006 — Grand Livre du mois 2006 — Flammarion, 2005

Tantra de Kalachakra, Le Livre de la sagesse, « Traité du mandala », avant-propos du Dalaï-lama, texte intégral traduit du sanskrit, DDB, 2003

Kalachakra, guide de l'initiation et du guru yoga, enseignements du Dalaï-lama et de Jhado Rinpoché, DDB, 2002

L'Initiation de Kalachakra, texte intégral du rituel et enseignement du Dalaï-lama, DDB, 2001

Tantra de Kalachakra, Le Livre du corps subtil, préface du Dalaï-lama, texte intégral traduit du sanskrit, Grand Livre du mois 2001 — DDB, 2000

Enfants du Tibet, de cœur à cœur avec Jetsun Pema et sœur Emmanuelle, DDB, 2000

Books by Dr. Lionel Coudron

DR. LIONEL COUDRON is a physician with degrees in nutrition, acupuncture, biology, traumatology, sports medicine, and EMDR psychotherapy. He has also been teaching yoga for more than thirty years. As the cofounder of the Association "Médecine et Yoga," he was president of the French Federation of Hatha Yoga school of teachers from 2000 to 2004, and he now teaches in various schools training people to become yoga teachers. He has also written numerous reference books on yoga and health.

Books in French

Yoga — Bien vivre ses émotions Edition Odile Jacob, Paris, 2007

La Yogathérapie Edition Odile Jacob, Paris, 2010

Yogathérapie — Soigner le stress Editions Odile Jacob, Paris, 2013

Yogathérapie — Soigner l'insomnie Edition Odile Jacob, Paris, 2013

Yogathérapie — Soigner l'hypertension artérielle par le yoga Edition Odile Jacob, Paris, 2014

Yogathérapie — Soigner les troubles digestifs par le yoga Edition Odile Jacob, Paris, 2014

About the Authors

PHAKYAB RINPOCHE is a ranking lama and a highly renowned practitioner in the Gelugpa order of Tibetan Buddhism. In 1994, Rinpoche was recognized by the Dalai Lama to be the eighth reincarnation of the Phakyab Rinpoche, a venerated Buddhist teacher and healer who first awoke in the eleventh century. Rinpoche is instrumental in the development of international research protocols on therapeutic benefits of meditation. He teaches regularly at centers in Europe, the United States, Asia, and South America and speaks frequently around the world.

SOFIA STRIL-REVER, a Sanskrit scholar and a writer, is the French biographer of the Dalai Lama, with whom she wrote three books that have been translated into more than twenty languages. She is also cowriter of the film *Dalai Lama: Une vie après l'autre* [*Life After Life*] and coauthor of several books with Sister Emmanuelle. In India she received traditional training from an Indian pandit at the Central University for Tibetan Studies in Sarnath and from a Tibetan lama at the Kirti Monastery in Dharamsala. She completed the first-ever translation of the Buddhist scriptures of Kalachakra from Sanskrit into a Western language. Sofia Stril-Rever teaches meditation and mantra yoga. She gives numerous lectures and recitals of sacred mantras and has sung for the Dalai Lama, the Indian saint Amma, and the Hindu sage Sri Tathata.

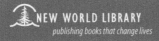